The Incontinence Diet

By

Lynne D M Noble

Wild River Health Publishing is committed to producing clear, accessible, and evidence-informed educational materials that support understanding, confidence, and practical wellbeing. Our focus is on bridging scientific knowledge with real-world experience, ensuring that readers of all backgrounds can engage with complex topics in a meaningful and empowering way.

We believe that health education should be grounded in clarity, compassion, and respect for the lived realities of individuals and communities. Every title we publish reflects this ethos, combining scientific insight with a commitment to dignity, autonomy, and lifelong learning.

We are proud to support authors who share these values and who strive to make knowledge both usable and humane.

About the Author

Lynne Noble, BSc (Hons), MSc, is a retired nutritional medicine practitioner, educator, and internationally published health writer. Her academic background includes a biomedical science–focused honours degree with study in genetics, immunology, Human Nutrition, pharmacology, and human physiology, alongside a Master's degree in Education specialising in science-based subjects.

She has completed postgraduate study in neurodegeneration and holds a **Diploma in Mental Health (Distinction)** and a **Diploma in Nutritional Medicine (Distinction) as well as research based experience in the field of statins and cholesterol**, in addition to numerous counselling and teaching qualifications. She has received multiple academic awards for her work and was nominated for the **Yorkshire Television Women of Achievement Award for Outstanding Academic Achievement**.

Lynne has taught at both college and university level, bringing clarity and compassion to complex subjects such as chronic illness, ageing, and environmental health. Her writing blends scientific insight with lived experience, empowering readers to understand their bodies and navigate complex healthcare systems with confidence.

A former member of the Guild of Health Writers and a member of the British Union of Journalists, she has written widely on nutrition, chronic disease, and patient experience. Her work champions dignity, understanding, and the human story behind every clinical label.

Contents

Preface

I had a number of subjects in my head to write in the future and this initially was not one of them even though we are now besieged by adverts urging people with incontinence problems to buy their (very expensive products), so that the problem is very difficult to ignore.

At the moment the problem of incontinence, and its solution, appears to be fixed on post pregnancy and sometimes older women go into raptures because certain incontinence pants address their issues. Or does it?

Does the prospect of spending a large fortune, which could be spent on cruises or landscaping the garden, really appeal? This is a lifelong – so we are informed – problem.

Those who went down the 'mesh route' are in crippling pain. There are law suits out. Is there not a simpler way without all these intrusive procedures which rob of dignity?

Men also suffer incontinence problems but rarely talk about it. It is mainly a side effect of an operation for prostate cancer. Just as incontinence robs women of their femininity, incontinence   robs men of their masculinity.

While the voices of women are becoming more strident about this unforeseen imposition on their life, men often suffer in silence…… and suffer they do.

Only one man has told me about his incontinence issues and the pads he has to wear. He says these are pretty useless as he cannot feel when his pads are wet and it often wets his clothing. This inability to feel was the side effect of his operation for a prostate problem. I wonder if nutritional medicine had been tried first.

There is stress incontinence and urge incontinence. There is the incontinence that can occur during the night when you sit up to go to the toilet (for the second time) and gravity is a little stronger than your muscles.

Of course, there is always advice such as 'Drink less before you go to bed (what if you are thirsty) or do Kegel's. (I know of no-one where this has actually worked) or perhaps a medicine like Ditropan may help – more about Ditropan and its dangers later.

Did anyone thing that this may be a nutritional issue? Perhaps not because we have been led away by the 'experts' into the intrusive world of medicine and mesh and the profiteering of pads in all shapes, sizes and colours.

We have done so willingly because we have been told that there is no other option. Our muscles are damaged (really?) and our prostates are shot (eye roll) or this is 'age-related' and we must just learn to live with it, except the ageing process is not a stage of chronic pain or incontinence even though that myth abounds. Ageing does not include that, it is a lie that has been put into people's minds as this book will show you.

Firstly, we will look at the different forms of urinary incontinence along with their definitions.

Although this book is primarily about urinary incontinence, I shall include bowel incontinence in and amongst.

The forms of urinary incontinence

Urinary incontinence is the accidental leakage of urine and has a number of causes which need to be addressed. These are:

The over active bladder which appears to afflict women who have had babies or are female and elderly.

An overactive bladder often means that those affected do not go out without planning where the toilets are on their journey. They may frequently visit every toilet, regardless of whether they need it at that particular time 'just in case.'

To understand what is happening, we need to learn a little about the bladder – an organ which is in the lower abdomen. Most people are not really aware of where it is, until they get a urinary infection and then they have a quick lesson in exactly where it is placed.

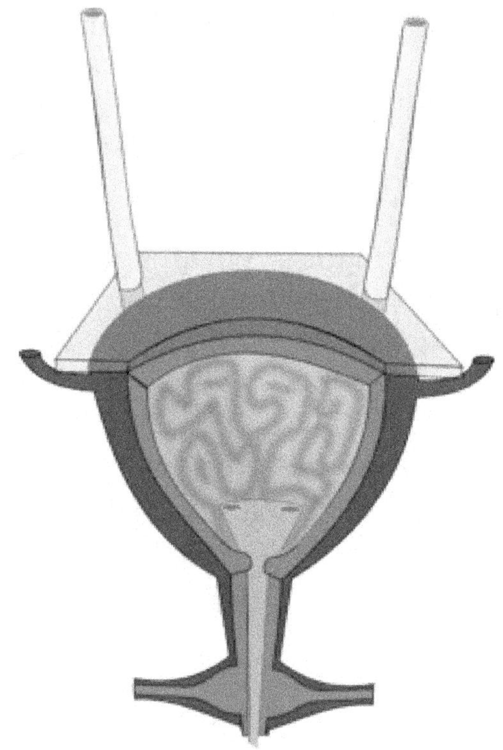

Simple diagram of the bladder, urethra and ureters

The bladder is a hollow organ with a great deal of elasticity in it. It forms part of the urinary system which also includes the:

Kidneys

Ureters

Urethra

Where the ureters are the two tubes attaching the kidneys to the bladder and the urethra is the single tube below the bladder.

When urination occurs, muscles tighten the bladder to enable it to move urine into the urethra and concurrently, the muscles surrounding the urethra relax to allow the urine to move out of the body.

Sometimes the synchronisation of this process falters allowing urinary leakage or incontinence.

When we look at the reasons for urinary incontinence, they are manifold and include:

Urinary tract infections

Vaginal infection or irritants like soap or 'over washing.'

Some medications or beverages like coffee which is a known irritant

Constipation

Damage to nerves due neurodegeneration, for example

Overactive bladder muscles

Pelvic organ prolapses (this is when the pelvic organs such the uterus, rectum and bladder move to a different place and press on the vagina or rectum.

obesity

Nutrient deficiencies (never investigated)

Men have different problems generally related to the prostate gland and include:

Damage to the prostate during surgery

Prostatitis – inflammation of the prostate gland

An enlarged prostate gland which may result in a condition known as benign prostate hyperplasia

There are different types of urinary incontinence. Stress incontinence occurs when stress is placed on the bladder such as you would find when:

Coughing

Sneezing

Laughing

Exercising

Or carrying something heavy

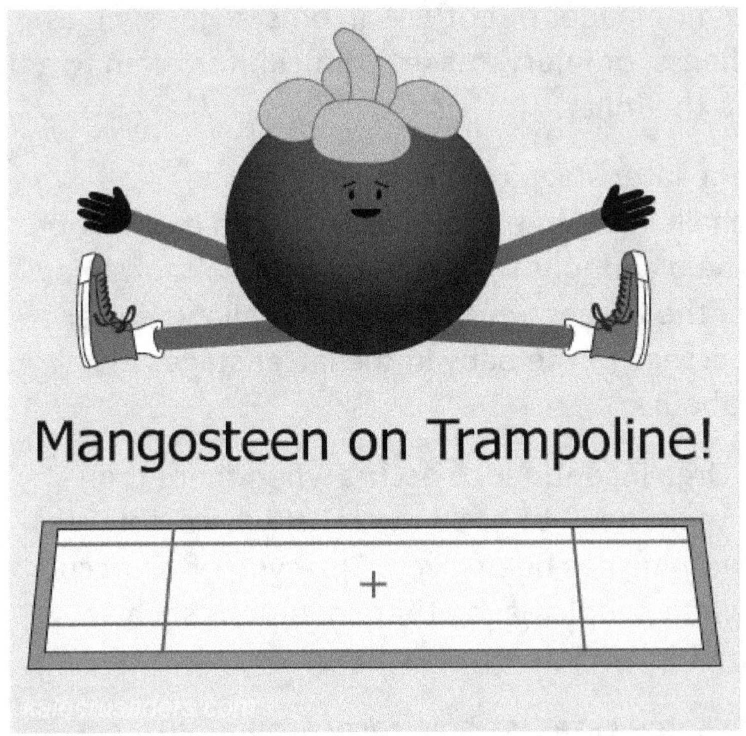

The majority of people with stress incontinence would find trampolining a challenge.

This type of incontinence can occur post pregnancy and during the menopause.

Functional incontinence occurs when the individual has absolutely nothing wrong with their bladder but other circumstances such as illness, or injury, make it difficult for them to get to the toilet.

The later stages of pregnancy can be challenging due to the baby's head pressing on the bladder as well as the hormonal 'softening' of the tissues which occurs and allows easier passage of the baby in the latter stages of labour.

Urge incontinence occurs when there is an urgent need to go to the toilet where not much warning has been given. This type often occurs when people have other conditions such as multiple sclerosis or diabetes.

In some cases, people carry around 'Just can't wait' cards to show people who may be in front of them in the toilet queue.

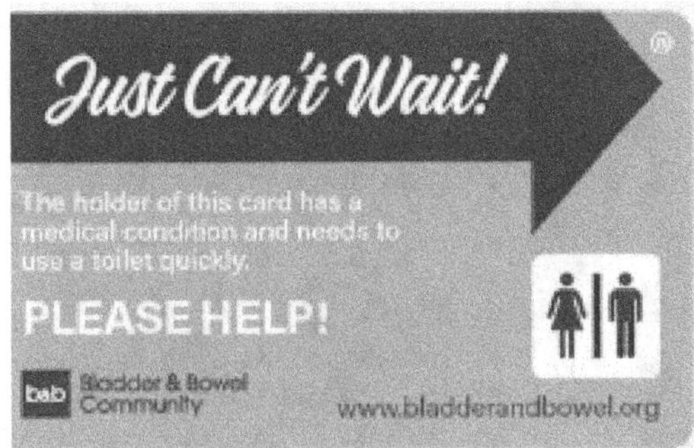

This is probably not helpful if the person in front is also carrying a 'just can't wait' card.

It is one of my bug bears that all toilets cannot cater for disabled people. If you have ever been waiting for a disabled toilet to become empty when the previous user needs at least half an hour to see to their needs, you will understand what I mean.

The practice of supermarkets leaving disabled toilets 'out of action' for prolonged periods needs challenging for this is becoming an increasingly common problem.

Overflow incontinence occurs due to leakage when the bladder is permanently full. This tends to occur in men if an enlarged prostate is blocking the urethra and is preventing the proper emptying of the bladder.

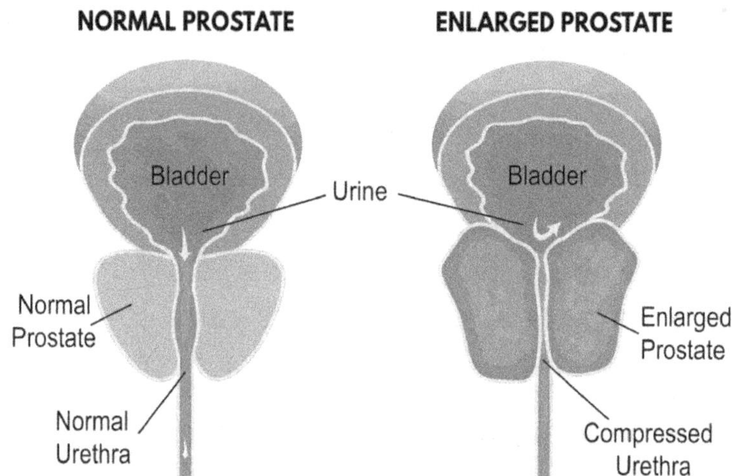

Here you can see how the enlarged prostate compresses the urethra preventing proper emptying of the bladder.

However, the neuropathy which accompanies diabetes or a spinal cord injury may also cause urinary leakage as the proper signals are not being relayed to the brain; these signals are needed to tell the bladder that it needs emptying.

As you can see there are a lot of things to consider when it comes to urinary incontinence as it does not have one cause. At this point it seems a natural progression to look at some of the above causes and some of the possible solutions to urinary incontinence.

As there are not many books addressing the subject of men's incontinence we will begin with this first. As most incontinence is due to an enlarged prostate, we will begin with that.

The enlarged prostate gland

The prostate is a small gland which is nestled deep within the groin between the base of the penis and the rectum.

It produces the semen which eventually is mixed with the sperm from the testes.

Benign enlargement of the prostate may occur in some men which is deemed to be part of the 'ageing process.'

In practice, as we shall see, it is no such thing and occurs as part of a nutrient deficiency. However, if benign enlargement does occur you would expect to see these symptoms:

Dribbling or inability to urinate (urinary retention)

Incontinence

Pain with blood due to infection

Incomplete emptying of the bladder

Needing to get up frequently (more than twice) during the night to empty the bladder

Sometimes the person has to strain to pass urine or there is a delayed start to the action of passing urine.

The symptoms of prostate cancer are very similar. The treatment of prostate cancer can lead to devastating and life long side effects.

Simon's story

In 2021, I was diagnosed with prostate cancer. I was informed that I would need an operation and I underwent this shortly after fully believing I would get rid of the problem and I would be able to lead a normal life after.

The reality is far different. After the operation I found I was incontinent. I have no feeling down there and do not know when I need to go to the toilet. I have to wear men's incontinence pants which is embarrassing, and costly. As I don't know when the pad is full, there is often leakage anyway so I have stopped going out or interacting with the people and groups that I used to do as I often need to change my clothes. There is simply no way of knowing whether I have passed more urine than usual so unless I am checking every

half hour or so, then I am unaware of the leakage or the need to change clothing.

Prostate cancer often responds to alternative forms of treatment[1] while an enlarged prostate is often due to a zinc deficiency and responds very well to increased intake of food containing zinc and/or supplementation of zinc, bearing in mind that excess zinc will inhibit copper and iron. Therefore, if you are taking iron or copper supplements then they are better taken apart from any zinc supplements you might consider taking.

Zinc not only helps to reduce prostate enlargement but will, as a result, improve urine flow and bladder emptying. The nocturnal trips to the loo, will diminish or cease, arresting the mental fog and general fatigue that accompanies a poor night's sleep.

The importance of zinc can be understood when you realise that the cells surrounding the

---

[1] https://www.amazon.co.uk/dp/B0C122VJ9P

prostate contain more zinc – up to 15 times more – than other somatic tissues.

Zinc is also required for the synthesis of testosterone. As age progresses an enzyme, - 5-alpha-reductase - converts testosterone to a substance called dihydrotestosterone (DHT) which is the degraded product.

The result of this is that an imbalance between the hormone testosterone and the hormone oestrogen occurs. It is this imbalance that begins the process of the enlargement of the prostate.

Now zinc deficiency has been found to impede the liver's ability to degrade steroid hormones, the result of which would allow a greater conversion of oestrogen from testosterone.

As well as reducing prostate enlargement, zinc supplementation was able to regulate gene expression. Indeed, when zinc was presented to cells from a prostate showing enlargement, apoptosis (cell suicide) occurred.

Further, optimum levels of zinc may protect from prostate cancer.

A 2011 study[2] has provided evidence of zinc's protective properties in this matter where it was found that those with lower levels of zinc were more likely to have BPH.

The recommended intake (RDI) of zinc is woefully low and even then is rarely reached.

In the UK it is 11mg for men and 9mg for women.

In the US it is 15mg

The recommended amount for prostate problems is 30mg once or twice daily to be taken with meals.

Zinc Picolinate is the preferred choice.

The use of proton pump inhibitors, like Omeprazole, will prevent the absorption of zinc.

---

1. [2] Christudoss P, Selvakumar R, Fleming JJ, Gopalakrishnan G. "Zinc status of patients with benign prostatic hyperplasia and prostate carcinoma." *Indian Journal of Urology: Journal of the Urological Society of India.* 2011;27(1):14-18.

and the use of diuretics like Furosemide will flush zinc out of your system rapidly.

As it is the body only stores a 24-hour supply of zinc.

Good sources of zinc are all animal proteins. While some zinc can be found in a plant based diet, it is not bioavailable due to the anti-nutrients in the plants. In this case it is the phytates which bind to zinc prevent its absorption.

The practice of replacing cow's milk with plant based milks would be a risk factor for sub optimal zinc levels.

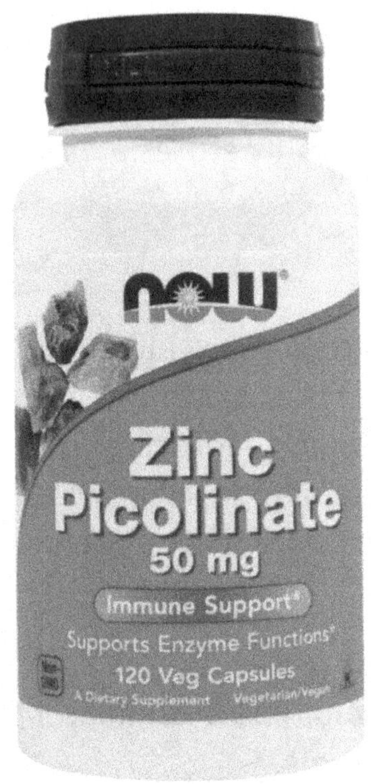

Vitamin D is also able to prevent excessive growth of the stromal and epithelial cells found in BPH. It is the excessive growth of these cells that produce the symptoms of BPH.

BPH is common; current numbers are believed to be about 50% of the male population and by the time   the man has reached the age of 80 years, it is likely that on average, only 10% will have escaped this condition.

This should not really surprise us given that both vitamin D deficiency (as well as zinc deficiency) are rife in society.

BPH is not generally a condition which affects younger men. It tends to affect older people because primarily because absorption of nutrients is poorer and the amount of food ingested decreases as appetite decrease. How often do we hear people say?

'I can't eat as much as I used to. I used to be able to eat a horse and now if I so much as look at something, I put a stone on.'

A review was undertaken to compile all the relevant data on any correlation between Vitamin D and BPH. Once this was completed it was incorporated into a complete article.

The results showed that vitamin D had an inhibitory effect on a pathway known as the ROCK pathway. (Rhoa) as well as;

Prostaglandin E2 expression and

BPH stromal cells

Where the Rock pathway is involved in cellular growth.

Stromal cells are tissues surrounding the epithelium surrounding the prostate. It is composed mainly of smooth muscle but contains blood vessels and nerves among some immune system cells

It was noted that increasing vitamin D through diet or supplementation reduced the prevalence of BPH.

The dosage used to decrease the volume of the prostate is 6000IU's daily. This should be compared to the miniscule 400iu's of vitamin D daily that is the Recommended Daily Intake.

 It is difficult enough to get 400 IU's of vitamin D daily in the diet, never mind 6000 IU's unless you live in a permanently sunny climate.

Reassuringly, all the studies have not noted any negative impact from the increased vitamin D in spite of general, but unsubstantiated warnings, in the general domain, that more than 400 IU's daily could be harmful.

I shall turn the attention from problems that just relate to male urinary incontinence to more general responses which would apply to both males and females. For example, urinary tract infections are common to both although women, due to their shorter urethra, have an increased likelihood of infection. After all, bacteria do not have as far to travel before colonising the bladder.

We shall look at the subject of infection later but at the moment I intend to look at two nutritional deficiencies which are involved with an overactive bladder.

We shall continue with that of vitamin D3 as its impact on urinary incontinence is nowhere near finished.

Vitamin D3 and the overactive bladder

A journal article entitled 'Vitamin D levels and the risk of overactive bladder: a systematic review and meta- analysis (vole 2, issue 2, February 2024 investigate whether a vitamin D deficiency could contribute to an over active bladder or urinary incontinence

If vitamin D deficiency was a potential culprit, then would supplementation treat it?

706 articles relating to this were found in a literature research. 13 of these were included in the review. These included:

Case control studies

Randomised controlled trials

Cohort studies

Cross sectional studies

The conclusion drawn was there was an increased risk of overactive bladder and urinary incontinence.

The authors also note that,' on the basis of existing data, the risk of urinary incontinence was reduced by 66% after vitamin D supplementation.

Why does vitamin D treat overactive bladder?

Vitamin D receptors are found in every tissue and organ in the body and this includes the bladder.
Vitamin D can help overactive bladders in a number of ways
- Vitamin D is able to help fight urinary infections. It does this by inducing an antimicrobial peptide (amp) called cathelicidin in the bladder. Cathelicidin has a number of functions which include:
  a) Neutralising endotoxins
  b) Reducing inflammation

Any inflammatory process will irritate the bladder so increasing cathelicidin through vitamin D supplementation will be of benefit.

While saturated animal fat, fatty fish like mackerel, and irradiated mushrooms do contribute some vitamin D to the diet, it is not enough. Our greatest source would be the sun but this is often in short supply.

For vitamin D to be made in the skin, it requires cholesterol so cholesterol reducing medications like statins can disrupt this process.

Vitamin D needs fat for its absorption so people on low fat diets will not fare well.

Vitamin D also needs magnesium for its activation but both vitamin D and magnesium are found to be deficient in a high proportion of the population.

Even if you get enough vitamin D but not enough magnesium (and vice versa) then the whole process fails as it would if an individual was on a low fat diet.

Nutrients do not work in isolation from each other. Further, absorption tends to be more impaired as we age although that could be attributed to poorer diet for a number of reasons.

- The vitamin D receptors are to be found in the smooth muscle and the skeletal muscle of the bladder and pelvic floor. Without sufficient vitamin D, muscles can become over active, irritable and hyper-contractile. There is also benefits for the pelvic floor as the muscle strength is improved when there is sufficient vitamin D.

It can thus be seen that sufficient vitamin D is essential to good bladder functioning. However, other nutrient deficiencies can be implicated. One common deficiency especially as we age is that of vitamin B12 deficiency. It is to this that we shall turn our attention to now.

Vitamin B12 deficiency and it's link with incontinence.

The key points are:

- Vitamin B12 is a fairly common nutrient deficiency in older age which occurs for a number of reasons
- Vitamin B12 requires an acidic environment to be separated from the protein source it is attached to but stomach acidity tends to decrease as we age.
- The release of stomach acid requires sufficient thiamine (vitamin B1) to be present yet this is a common nutrient deficiency.
- Vitamin B12 is a water soluble vitamin and, as such is easily flushed out of the body. Diuretic use is very common post

menopause and these medications will contribute to vitamin B12 deficiency.

On the whole people tend to eat less red meat as they age; chewing can be a problem or general lack of interest can contribute. However, this is not a definitive list.

Vegan and vegetarian lifestyles contribute to the potential risk of vitamin B12 deficiency. Vitamin B12 is found in animal protein, not fruits and vegetables.

A study illustrates the relationship between vitamin B12 and incontinence.

Both men and women were involved in the study. The records show that the majority were women.

Both urinary and faecal incontinence were included.

The conclusion of the study was that vitamin B 12 deficiency was not linked to isolated urinary or faecal incontinence but there was an association with double incontinence.

However, as vitamin B12 is vital for the health of nerves, if nerve damage should occur then nervous transmission signalling when the bladder is full and needs emptying may not work well resulting in urinary incontinence

A single blood test can identify a vitamin B12 deficiency. However, there are a number of signs and symptoms which may alert you to such a deficiency. A yellowish tinge to the skin is one such sign. Others include:

- Fatigue
- Headaches
- Nausea
- Sore mouth or tongue
- diarrhoea
- weight loss

There are also neurological symptoms which include:

- numbness or tingling in the feet and hands
- balance problems

- confusion
- poor recall
- visual problems
- mood disorders

Other symptoms which may occur more rarely are:

- a smooth red tongue
- tinnitus (in both ears as this is a systemic disorder)
- feeling breathless, dizzy or faint

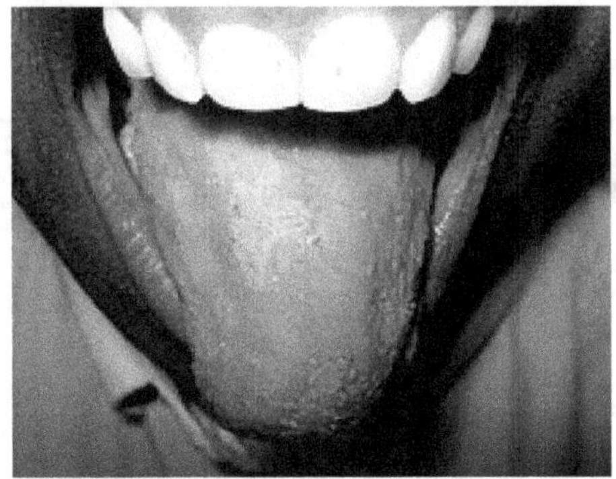

A smooth red tongue is a sign of vitamin B12 deficiency

Increasing vitamin B12 in the diet and attending to other potential deficiencies which may contribute should rectify the deficiency. In some cases, individuals still cannot absorb it and may need injections – which work rapidly – or, in some cases, there are sub-lingual lozenges which can be bought from health food shops. These can be placed below the tongue or between the upper lip and gum where it can be absorbed. This bypasses the stomach which is unable to absorb vitamin B12 due to a condition known as pernicious anaemia.

Years ago, before B12 injections were invented, individuals suffering from pernicious anaemia had to eat large amounts of raw liver, on a daily basis, in order to be able obtain enough vitamin B12 for their needs.

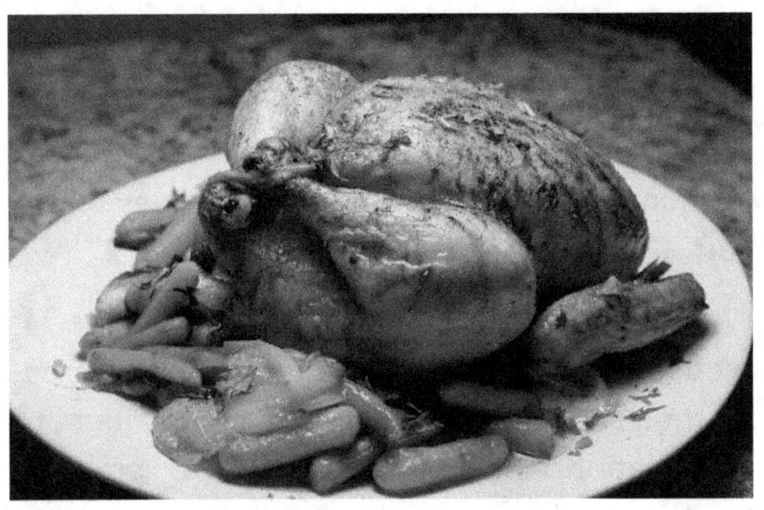

Roast chicken contains vitamin B12 unlike the accompanying vegetables.

B vitamins are water soluble and are not stored in the body. However, vitamin B12 is unusual in that it can and is stored in the body: up to two years' worth. Does this reflect its importance? The B vitamins – all of them – are vital to health.

Obesity, vitamin C deficiency and urinary incontinence

Urinary incontinence is indirectly linked to a vitamin C deficiency where obesity does play a part.

Where abdominal fat presses on the bladder, it reduces the volume of urine that can be stored. Further, such abdominal mass may contribute to constipation which can cause further pressure on the bladder. If the pressure is further increased by sneezing or coughing, then the results can be very distressing for the individual.

While studies evidencing that vitamin C is able to help urinary incontinence through direct mechanisms, it is able to reduce abdominal fat mass which may reduce pressure on the bladder. Further, adequate amounts of vitamin C is able to alleviate constipation with the negative impact of many popular and over the counter medications.

Vitamin C keeps fluid in the bowel which increases stool size, triggering a bowel movement, as well as making it easier to pass.

Further, vitamin C induces carnitine to fulfil its function.

Carnitine is a conditional amino acid which helps to carry fat into cells to be burned for energy. It appears to be especially successful in the abdominal area although this may not be noticeable for about 3 months and the vitamin C intake must be adequate.

Conditional means that the requirements for this substance outweigh the body's ability to synthesise it in the liver, brain and kidneys.

The amino acids methionine and lysine are essential to this process.

What are the main sources of the amino acid, carnitine?

The main sources are red meat especially followed by other protein sources. Some is found in plants but certainly not enough for the body's needs.

Carnitine's critical function is that of energy production. It fulfils this by helping transport long chain fatty acids into the mitochondria. These are tiny organelles found in all cells. There they are oxidised and this produces energy known as adenosine triphosphate (ATP).

Carnitine's further function is that it helps transport toxic waste out of the mitochondria.

Some tissues are more likely to oxidise carnitine than others. For example, the heart muscle and skeletal muscle are prime examples of tissues that require long chain fatty acids for their energy supply.

Long Chain Fatty Acids (LCFA'S) are those which are stored as adipose tissue, that is the 'fat' that most people are dieting to get rid of.

It is difficult to avoid LCFA's. They can be found in all vegetable oils as well as butter, cocoa, shea oils, among others.

They can be further divided into

Saturated and

Unsaturated fatty acids

Where the former is generally of animal origin with coconut oil being an exception as it is generally solid at room temperature.

Regardless of their source they seem inclined to store themselves around the abdomen.

A recommended daily intake is around 20mg with those on a carnivore diet generally exceeding this and those on a plant based diet not quite reaching this amount. However, some is made endogenously and that which isn't needed will be excreted.

Further, we should not forget that the synthesis of carnitine requires adequate vitamin C.

What do we mean by adequate? It is one of those. 'How long is a piece of string questions.'

The requirements for vitamin C differs widely between individuals so that some people may get by on 500mg daily whilst others may need 3000-4000mg daily

This is because vitamin C has many functions including helping he synthesis of collagen – a protein which forms the larger part of connective tissue like skin, tendons, ligaments. It is vital for the smooth ticking over of the immune system, alleviating mood disorders, as it help make hormones and countless other functions which rarely get a mention.

This means that daily requirements very much depend on what is going on in the body. Feel stressed? This increases the need for vitamin C.

The best way of trying to figure out what is a likely amount of vitamin C that is specific to your requirements, is to take the bowel tolerance test by increasing your intake of vitamin C by 1000mg every hour. Once the body's tissues are saturated then the bowel releases its contents quite rapidly and easily.

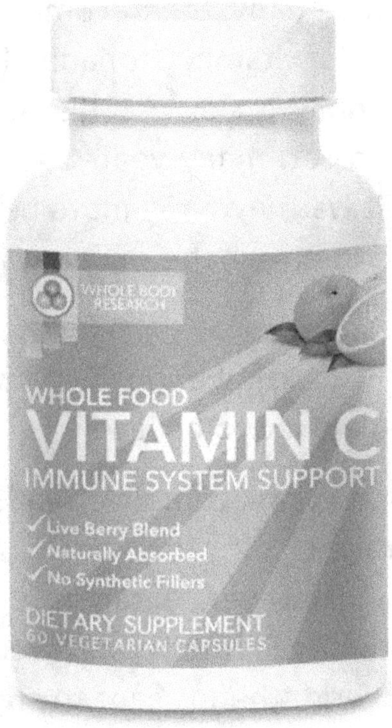

Although I would like to say that adequate vitamin C is obtainable from the diet, it is becoming increasingly apparent that vitamin C deficiency is increasing and may need supplementation.

Do not be fooled by the recommended daily intake of 75mg of vitamin C for adult females and 90mg for adult males. This is laughably miniscule, and set, many years ago, to prevent scurvy only. It was never meant to be an amount that resulted in any shape or form, in optimum health overall.

It is more difficult to get enough vitamin C in your diet than you are led to believe.

A medium orange will contain about 30mg if it is plucked straight off the bush and eaten immediately. However, vitamin C dissipates rapidly in storage. Fruit that travels half way around the world, then is sent to supermarkets where it may languish for some time, is unlikely to have much, if any, vitamin C left. Therefore, the exhortation to eat 'five a day' or '10 a day' may provide other nutrients which do not suffer degradation but it is unlikely to contain any vitamin C of merit.

Vitamin C is destroyed by heat. Cooking virtually eliminates it. Even the shortest steaming will reduce the vitamin C content to next to nothing.

When families used to grow their own, post war, the food was picked just prior to it being eaten. Proud husbands and fathers grew copious amounts of tomatoes in their greenhouse, picked lettuces from their land and plucked fruit straight from the tree at the time it was going to be eaten. Now, that was an example of vitamin C from land to table in a way that preserved it for eating.

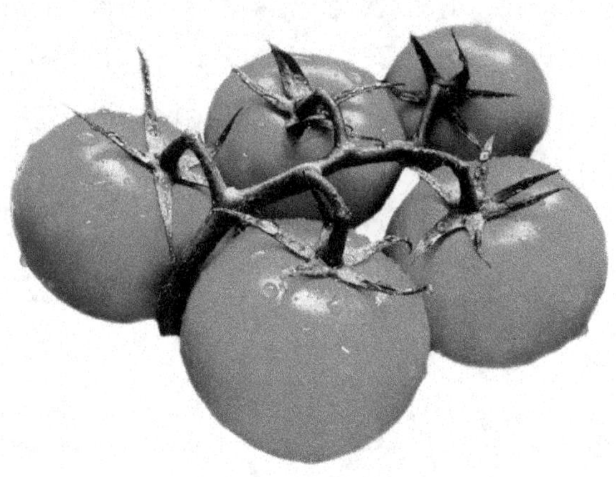

Home-grown tomatoes will contain vitamin C.

In the 1950's people used to make their own rose hip syrup. Rose hips are full of vitamin C but the actual preparation probably destroyed it all leaving a sweet syrupy pink liquid designed to increase blood sugar levels dramatically.

Rose hip syrup requires a lot of simmering to extract the flavour but it is this process that destroys the vitamin C.

Currently, vitamin C deficiency is the fourth most common deficiency in the United States.

Our fast food lifestyle has probably done much to fuel the increase in urinary incontinence in a number of ways. Firstly, there is little or no vitamin C in fast food so carnitine's function is impeded; fat will build up.

Fast food is highly calorific and is a risk factor for obesity.

Vitamin C enhances the function of thiamine which enhances the function of vitamin B12. As you have probably gathered by now, no nutrient works in isolation. It will impact the work of other specific nutrients and, in turn, be impacted by them. A deficiency of one which is not directly involved in a process can still prevent another that is, from optimum efficacy.

An example of this is the impact of vitamin C on thiamine. People who lack thiamine almost certainly will retain fluid in the lower limbs. This is generally removed from the tissues when the individual is lying down at night. This can result in a frequently interrupted sleeping pattern due to numerous trips to the toilet.

When the heart is functioning properly then it will remove excess fluid efficiently during the day. Night time trips to the toilet are an indication that a person's nutritional intake needs to be looked at.

Night time incontinence is tiring and disruptive.

Vitamin C does help thiamine's function. However, lack of vitamin C, can in itself, be a risk factor for heart failure.

Vitamin C and histamine

Some unfortunate people tend to have higher levels of histamine than the majority of the population. These unfortunates will no doubt have other allergic type conditions such as asthma, eczema, persistently stuffy nose and hay fever.

When the deeper layers of tissue are involved we refer to this as angioedema. Many people will be familiar with this in relation to peanuts where these are alleged to cause full blown anaphylaxis.

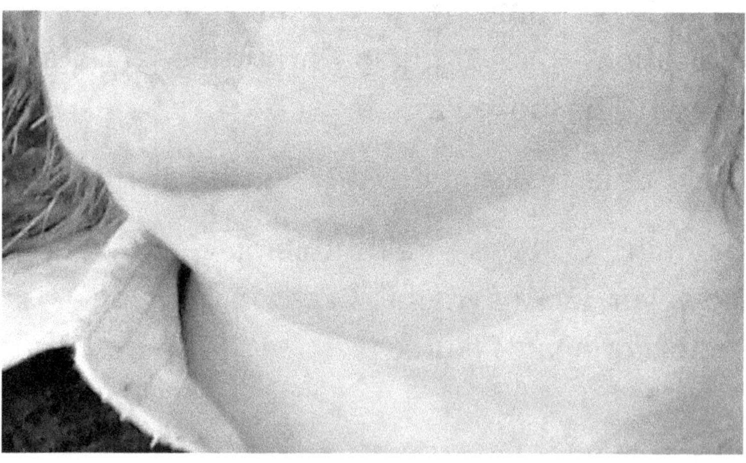

Beginning of angioedema where the throat is just beginning to swell. A full blown attack will require the administration of an epipen.

Histamine irritates the sensitivity of bladder nerves as it will do with any other nerves it comes into contact with. Irritation is generally followed by a localised oedema. We have two risks for urinary incontinence here; irritated, sensitive bladders and extra pressure.

Antihistamines may be suggested since they block the function of histamine receptors but they have numerous other negative side effects including weight gain and an increased risk for dementia if taken over the long term. Drowsiness is a very common side effect.

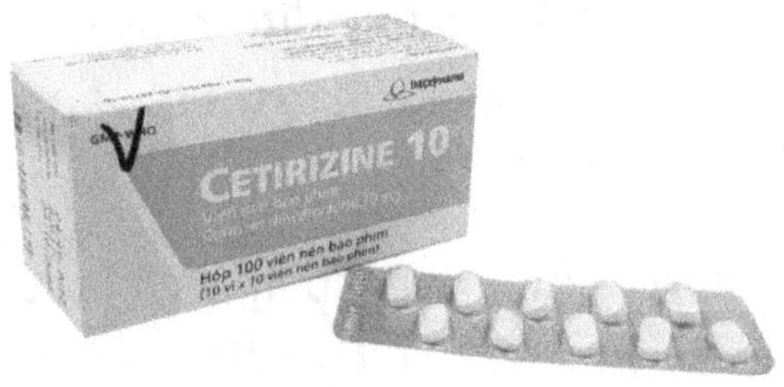

Cetirizine is a   common antihistamine which could be used as a sleeping aid as it has marked soporific effects

Vitamin C works in a different way by reducing the synthesis of histamine. It is equally, if not more effective than antihistamines and without the side effects, including drowsiness. Indeed, as vitamin C is needed to induce carnitine to transport fat into cells for burning energy, then it increases energy and alertness.

Vitamin C deficiency is known as scurvy and many people live sub optimally with this condition. It is rarely tested for as it generally goes unrecognised. It may take up to 3 months for this condition to be addressed through proper supplementation of vitamin C. However, there will be subtle positive differences from day one such as increased alertness and better balance.

Any bladder dysfunction such as bladder pain syndrome or interstitial cystitis which causes, frequency, pain or urgency should be treated with vitamin C before attempting prescription medications.

Vitamin C is cheap, has other positive side effects and, as a water soluble vitamin, cannot be overdosed upon. Any excess vitamin C that the body cannot use will simply be flushed out of the body.

Once the underlying deficiency is corrected than those who are obese tend to start losing small amounts of weight weekly. Whether this is due to the extra energy and movement this affords, or carnitine's fat burning properties, or both, is anyone's guess. Rarely, dramatic weight loss has occurred but this may be more to do with the antihistamine properties of vitamin C since it then prevents fluid build-up in tissues.

Oedematous tissues can result in over a stone in extra weight.

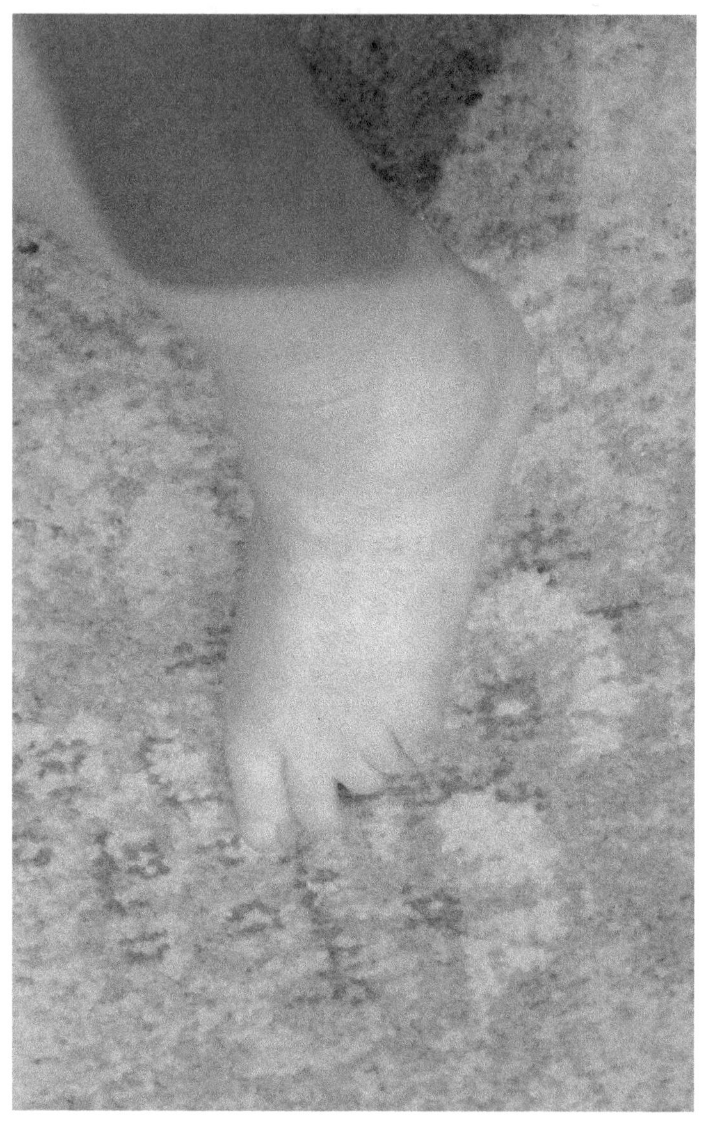

Fluid build-up in tissues can increase weight dramatically but responds to optimum amounts of vitamin C and thiamine.

Food items which contain high levels of histamine are spinach, anything with vinegar added such as pickled beetroot, tomatoes and tinned foods.

Indirectly, stress may also result in urinary incontinence where anxiety ridden people are visiting every toilet that they know of 'just in case.'

This results in them voiding very small amounts so that the bladder, which is elastic and strong and can hold up to 500ml of urine will never be used to full efficacy. Eventually, it is 'trained' to want to void at quarter capacity.

Most people will make a trip to void the bladder at around 150ml. It is easy to see what your capacity is by peeing into a jug which can measure the amount.

It would not surprise most people that the amount is probably less than 150ml, especially if they are adult females.

The good news is that you can retrain the bladder to feel comfortable at more than 150ml's although if you eat or drink an irritant such chilli or coffee that the bladder may want to void at small amounts.

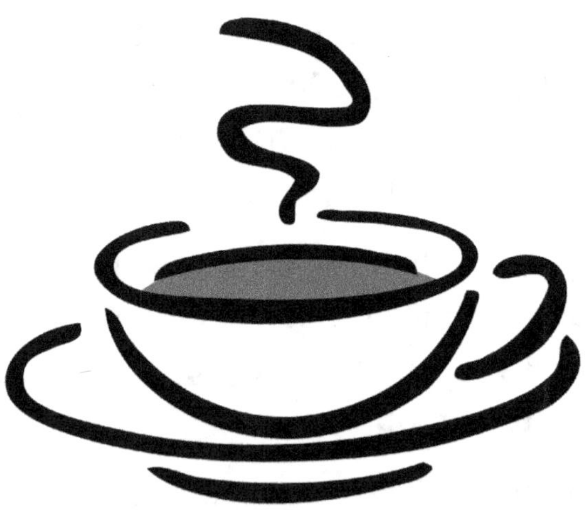

Coffee is a bladder irritant

Benfotiamine

Benfotiamine is the synthetic form of thiamine and has the added advantage of being fat soluble with a better ability to enter cells.

Benfotiamine is useful in that helps with weight loss.

Originally, it was investigated for its impact on controlling blood sugar levels. Thiamine is known for its antidiabetic effects as it is needed to push glucose into the cells to be burnt for energy. Benfotiamine was thought it may do this better than naturally occurring water soluble thiamine as it was able to enter cell better.

Later, it was found to promote weight loss in those who were overweight or obese. While the weight loss was not dramatic, it was still significant.

Alongside vitamin C supplementation, glucose and fat is burned for energy. Occurs with the aid of benfotiamine   thus promoting weight loss, reducing abdominal obesity and helping reduce the pressure on the bladder caused by this internal fat.

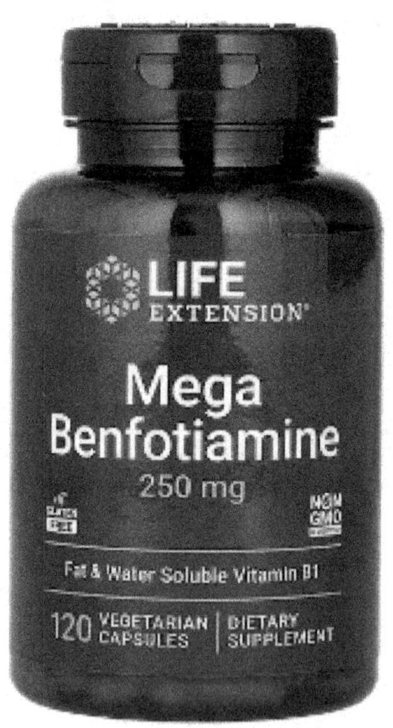

Benfotiamine can help in weight reduction.

Magnesium and incontinence issues.

Magnesium is an abundant mineral in the body required for approximately 300 reactions in the body including activating vitamin D and thiamine. Magnesium deficiency can not only directly urinary incontinence but indirectly affect this condition by rendering vitamin D and B1 inactive.

Some of its other functions include:

Muscle/nerve function

Protein synthesis

Regulating blood pressure

Regulation of blood sugar

Reduction of spasm and contributes to normal heart rhythm

The majority of magnesium is found in the bones and the rest apart from about 1% is found soft tissues. The 1% found in serum is hard to measure, so magnesium is not routinely tested for; it hardly evidences whether there is sufficient in the soft tissue or bone. This would require different tests, the cost of which are likely prohibitive.

The kidneys help regulate the amount of magnesium in the system.   When there is a deficiency of magnesium then urinary excretion is low. Magnesium supplements, in the absence of a deficiency could potentially increase urination.

Magnesium's anti-spasmodic properties may help with irritable bladders.

Similarly, calcium is also associated with an overactive bladder and nocturia (night voiding)) as well as nocturnal polyuria (excessive urine production).

If excessive calcium excretion should occur, then at night time the amount of antidiuretic hormone that is secreted, is reduced. Antidiuretic hormone concentrates the urine at night so that you are not constantly getting up; calcium disrupts this.

Many elderly people are routinely given calcium supplements by their GP's. While osteoporotic bones may be caused by many nutrients deficiencies, including vitamin C and zinc, the poor absorbable form of calcium is routinely prescribed. How much this contributes to the frequent night time trips to the toilet is not known but it is a consideration.

In any event, withdrawing the supplement for a few days will help establish whether calcium is the culprit. If it is, remember that it is excessive calcium that is being excreted not the calcium that the body needs to keep it ticking over in optimum health.

Calcium supplementation is heavily promoted. Calcium is already hidden in bread, added to soy milk and medications for indigestion. It is also added to breakfast cereals which is probably counterproductive since it is not an absorbable form of calcium.

Further, calcium needs to be taken little and often; that is the only way that it can be absorbed. There is no point in adding a whole days recommended daily intake in a bowlful of cereal and believe that it is all going to be absorbed.

Calcium carbonate is, after all, chalk. This form of calcium also requires an acidic stomach for it to be absorbed; this is something that elderly people are less likely to have.

Acidity appears to reduce as ageing occurs. Post menopause can be tricky where women blame shrinking tissues for their urinary problems. The exhortation to supplement with calcium to take care of bones is not considered as a potential reason for their new found urinary issues.

Other well-known sources of calcium are:

Yogurt

Milk

Cheese

nuts

These form a large part of people's diets.

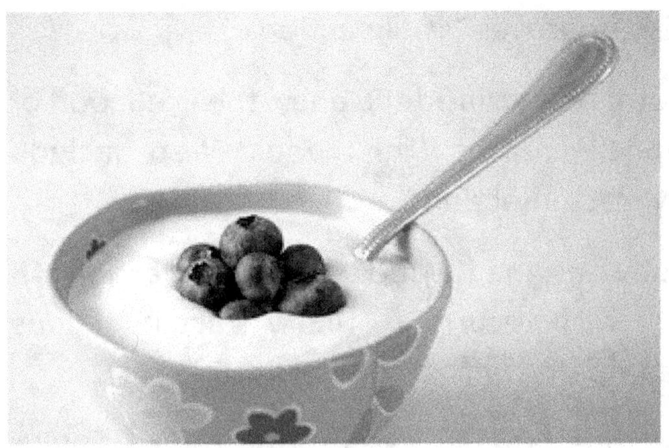

Yogurt is a good source of calcium but too much calcium can be a risk factor for nocturia and nocturnal polyuria.

The zinc connection to urinary problems

Zinc is an essential trace mineral. It is highly concentrated in the body in healthy individuals and is present in every cell in the body.

It has a multiplicity of functions including:

- The breakdown of carbohydrates
- Cell division and cell growth
- Wound healing
- Sense of smell and taste

Zinc also improves insulin action

Where there is a zinc deficiency, the likelihood of infection increases; this would also include urinary tract infections.

In a study designed to look at this connection, 48 patients with recurring urinary tract infections were compared with a control group.

It was noted that levels of zinc reduced with ageing but overall levels of zinc were lower than those of the control group and lower zinc levels were a risk factor for urinary infection.

Diet will have a bearing on zinc levels. Animal proteins are good sources of zinc with shellfish the best of all sources.

Reasonable sources of zinc are whole grains, legumes, nutritional yeast and nuts. However, any food item which is plant based will contain anti nutrients –phytates – will grab hold of zinc so that it cannot be absorbed.

As it is, plant based diets and low protein diets may be a risk factor for infections of any kind.

Once a zinc deficiency occurs it tends to be self-perpetuating as one of the side effects is reduced appetite. As well as poor appetite, loss of hair is an indicator.

It can be seen that many of the accepted characteristics of older age are nothing but nutritional deficiencies. That is:

Thinning hair

Loss of smell and taste

Poor appetite.

Poor wound healing

Repeated infections

A simple blood test for zinc deficiency could be undertaken but rarely is by GP's. The better way forward is to consider the symptoms of a deficiency and see if they improve with an improved diet or zinc supplementation.

The Recommended Daily Intake is said be around 11mg daily but this appears to be far too low in the light that, should a cold appear to be coming on, then 25mg-50mg is recommended.

Apart from low protein and plant based diets, diuretics – another medication which appears to be foisted on the elderly to treat the symptoms and not the underlying cause of a problem – will remove just about all the zinc in the body.

There is only enough zinc stored in the body to last for 24 hours so we don't have massive reserves of this vital nutrient as it is. Diuretics will flush most, if not all of the zinc, out of the system.

Another popular medication which prevents absorption of zinc are the proton pump inhibitors (PPI's). Well known ones are Omeprazole and Lansoprazole. These PPI's treat reflux conditions.

It should be noted that reflux is not normally a life-long aberration of any individual; it comes on for a reason and it is no good masking the symptoms without addressing the underlying cause.

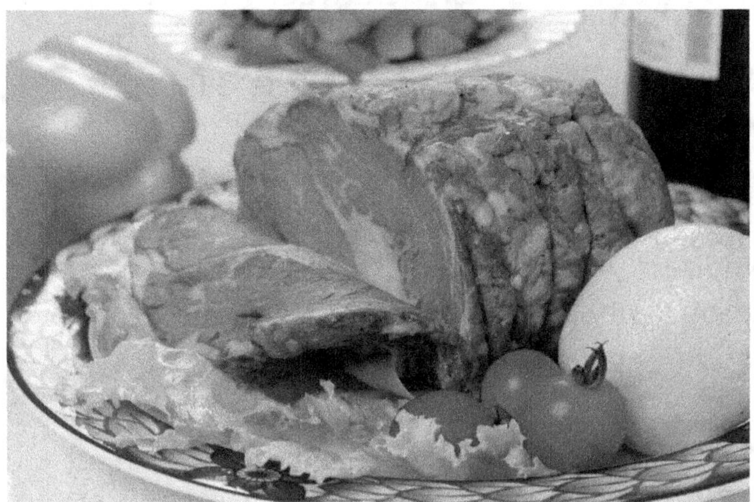

Beef is an excellent source of zinc

A zinc deficiency will also result in an enlarged prostate which creates problems for men and their urine flow. For those individuals who have followed my recommendations and increased zinc in their diet, they have been rewarded with a shrinking prostate with an easier flow of urine occurring at the same time.

There is also a relationship between zinc deficiency and abdominal obesity. Studies where the relationship between nutritional status, serum zinc levels and abdominal fat were investigated found that there is a positively significant correlation with abdominal fat.

Indirectly, zinc deficiency can impact a propensity to urinary incontinence through the additional pressure of abdominal fat.

Just as zinc deficiency can be implicated in pathological changes as ageing progresses, it is also true that ageing impacts zinc absorption.

While mastication is often a problem for some elderly – and this may reduce their desire for certain foods – milk and soft foods like cheese do contain zinc. Fish and minced meat are generally acceptable as are eggs.

It is worth totting up zinc intake for three or four days just to see if any adjustments to dietary intake needs to be made.

Four ounces of beef contain about 5.5mg

250ml milk contains about 1.2mg

Nuts contain zinc in varying amounts

A three ounce serving of oysters provide about 75mg. They are by far the best source of zinc. However, they are not a popular edition to most people's diets.

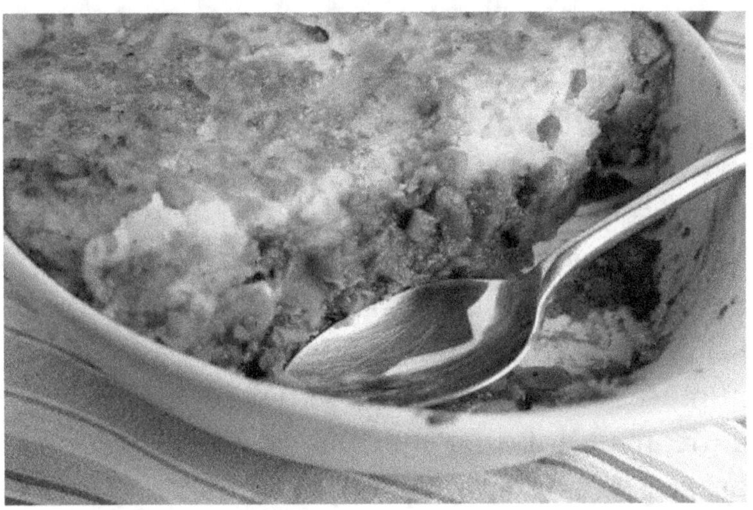

Cottage pie is a good way to get zinc in a form that is easy to eat. Minced beef is enjoyed by most people.

Bear in mind that when there is poor absorption then the 11mg that you think you are getting will probably only equate to about 5.5mg.

Elderly people should be aiming for about 20mg daily as should those with urinary conditions. It is not that easy to achieve as you would first think; well not unless you eat a lot of oysters.

Folate and urinary conditions

The nerves that innervate the urinary system require folate which you may be familiar with as folic acid, the synthetic form of folate.

In a research paper entitled, **Reversible central nervous system dysfunction in folate deficiency (E** Melamed, A Reches, C Hershko PMID: 1141959 an epileptic patient had numerous neurological disturbances due to the anticonvulsant drug she was on. These included progressive dementia and incontinence.

It was found, as is often the case with patients on anticonvulsant medications, that her serum folate levels were low. Following supplementation with folic acid, her symptoms, including the urinary incontinence resolved.

There are a number of causes of folate deficiency and these include:

- A diet which does not include enough foods which contain folate. These include, meat (liver is a good source), yeast products; nutritional yeast is excellent, green leafy vegetables, fortified cereals and fresh fruit. Fruit that has spent a long time on the shelf at the supermarket does not count.

- Alcohol depletes folate

- Conditions which affect the gastrointestinal tract such as Crohn's disease, coeliac disease, problems which require a stoma, operations to help reduce obesity, among others

- Other medications such as methotrexate which is commonly given to those with rheumatoid arthritis and similar conditions

- Pregnancy, so apart from the pressure on the bladder from the developing baby, the lower levels of folate may also contribute to the incontinence which mothers to be often suffer from.

- In some case, individuals have a mutation in the gene which prevents folate from being converted into its active form. They may need to take it in the form 5-methyl-THF.

The prevalence of this mutated genes does differ between races. For example, it is more prevalent in Hispanic people where one in four will have this mutation. In white and Asian people only one in ten are likely to have this mutated gene. This drops to one in a hundred in black people.

Folate deficiency can be ascertained by a single blood test.

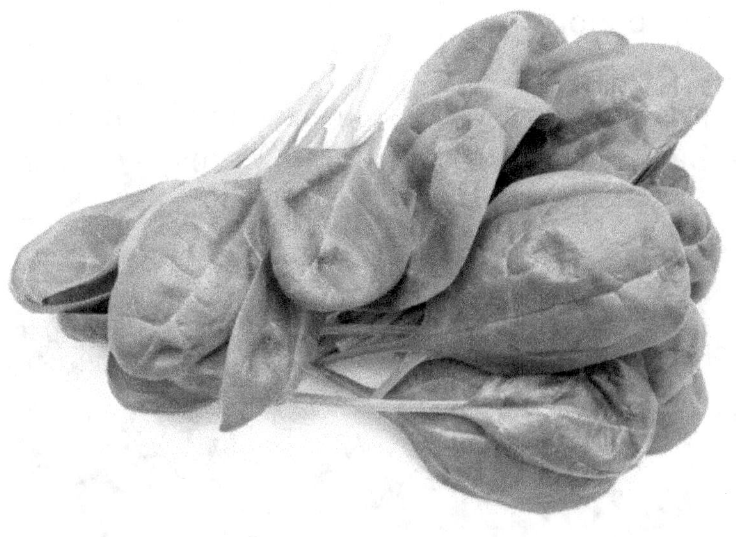

Spinach is a good source of folate as is any green leafy vegetable.

All in all, most urinary problems occur due to nutritional deficiencies which are a risk factor for:

Urinary tract infections

Obesity

Constipation

Minor irritation, will also has a bearing on our subject matter, may occur due to spices used in cooking especially those found in chilli and curries.

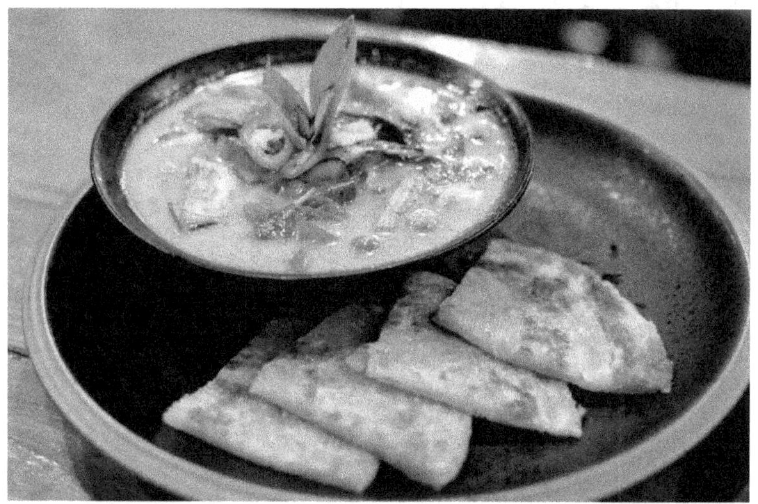

Spicy curry will irritate the bladder

While we are considering the fact that some food items may irritate the bladder, we also need to consider those other food and drink items which irritate the bladder and which we often ingest on a daily basis.

Food items which irritate the bladder

The most obvious foods which have the potential to irritate the bladder are those which have a high histamine content. Unfortunately, many foods contain histamine to some degree but as people have different histamine tolerance levels, many of the ones containing lower amounts need not be excluded if they are eaten in moderate amounts.

The foods to avoid in order to control histamine are:

- Ready meals

- Aged cheese

- Alcohol

- Yeast products

- Ripened or more mature foods are more likely to contain more histamine than their less mature counterparts.

- Pickled foods

- Fermenting foods such as yogurt and kefir

- Smoked meats

- Chocolate

- Legumes

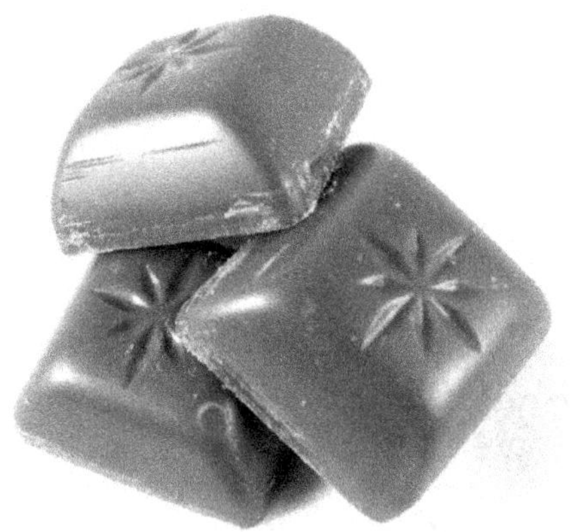

Chocolate can raise histamine levels

More acceptable foods are:

Chicken

Eggs

Fresh meat

Fresh fruit and vegetables but avoid
tomatoes which do have high levels; spinach
and eggplant are also to be avoided.

Grains like rice, white bread (no yeast) oats
and pasta are fine.

Fresh milk, cream cheese and butter are fine.

The enzyme diamine oxidase, which is found
in the kidneys, digestive tract and the
thymus, breaks down excessive histamine.
That is its prime function. However, certain
foods are known to block this enzyme so

that it cannot keep histamine levels down to acceptable ones.

These food and drink items are ones in common use and include:

Energy drinks

Black tea

Alcohol

Yeast (very high in DAO inhibitor)

On a personal note, I do have an intolerance to histamine but seemed to have avoided many food items which upset me, from an early age, without knowing why I was doing that. Nutritional yeast was one such popular item that my siblings ate with great relish but brought me out in hives. While I accepted the cod liver oil and rose hip syrup which were given on a daily basis, the malt made me feel ill and eventually I refused it.

'Faddy children' were not encouraged or tolerated in those times. Mother took it as a sign that her efforts to keep us healthy were not appreciated. Decades later I learned – after I had been issued with an Epipen for persistent facial and throat swelling – that 2g of vitamin C daily sorted the whole problem out. Note: the measly 75mg which is the daily amount recommended for vitamin C did not. Everyone has to find their own level.

Histamine makes skin leaky and oedematous such that if you write on your skin, the marks will remain.

Diamine Oxidase is found in kidney beans, peas and chickpeas. These are good sources for those with an intolerance to histamine.

While oleic acid (a component of olive oil) does not contain diamine oxidase, it does help to increase it in the blood.

Increasing foods which contain diamine oxidase, reducing intake of foods which block it and increasing vitamin C which naturally lowers histamine can make a huge difference to bladder irritation and incontinence.

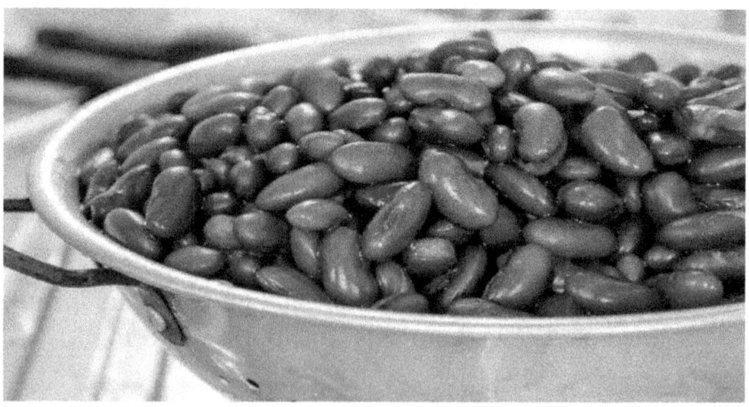

Kidney beans contain lots of diamine oxidase which helps break down histamine.

If changing the diet is too much then diamine oxidase can be purchased from health food shops to supplement your diet.

Onions have been used as a diuretic since Roman times; whether this is due to their potassium content, which helps balance water in and out of cells, or some other property has not been properly explored. Many other food items like melons have good amounts of potassium and while they are recognised as having a diuretic effect they do not enjoy the same lofty profile as onions for their impact on the bladder and bowel.

As tomatoes and other acidic foods like citrus are potential causes of irritable bladder, it is likely that the acid in onions contribute. However, onions contain allinase an enzyme that converts sulphoxides into sulphenic acid which is an irritant. Garlic will produce a similar result.

Once cooked, enzymes are easily destroyed and so the impact of the chemical reaction is nullified.

However, onions also contain citric, malic, oxalic and glutamic acids all of which give onions their unique flavour; these do not appear to be as problematical for irritating the bladder as sulphenic acid although citric acid, which is added to just about every processed food, comes a close contender.

Whilst the above nutritional deficiencies are more likely to contribute to incontinence, it is worth repeating that no nutrient works in isolation and, as such, a nutrient that is not directly involved may still have an effect. For example, folate deficiency has some impact on incontinence but the deficiency may not be due to poor intake but a lack of riboflavin which is required activate the folate.

There is no direct connection between riboflavin and problems with incontinence.

The menopause is another of those rites of passage that seem to be associated with bladder problems, so it may be useful to look at this now.

Menopause

What do people associate with the menopause?

Weight gain

Incontinence

Thinning hair

Mood swings

Wrinkles

Poor sleep quality

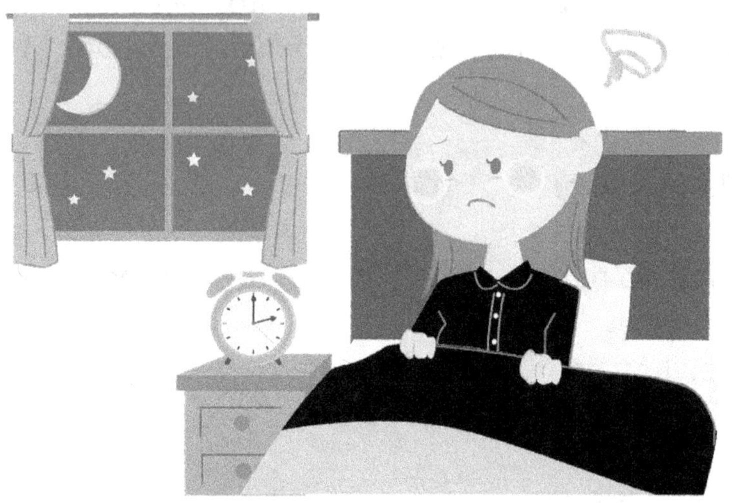

People associate insomnia with the menopause

In reality, all of the above symptoms could be attributed to a vitamin C deficiency.

Thinning of the skin, often put down to an oestrogen deficiency could well be due to lack of vitamin C. It is after all required in the synthesis of collagen so firm, plump tissue which functions well needs a good supply of it.

Thinning of the urethra is a risk factor for incontinence.

Vitamin C is also needed in the synthesis of hormones so it is reasonable to assume that decreasing oestrogen may also be due to insufficiency of vitamin C.

Oestrogen deficiency does need correcting as it can increase the risk for cardiovascular disease and atherosclerosis as well as bladder problems. There are two main ways that this can be achieved. Firstly, vitamin D is required for oestrogen metabolism so increasing your intake of vitamin D would help with thinning of the skin in the urethra.

How does vitamin D increase oestrogen levels?

Vitamin d helps modulate the enzymatic activity which converts androgens into oestrogens.

Vitamin D is able to influence gene expression. As we have already learned vitamin D receptors are found in every tissue and organ in the human body including reproductive tissues.

. Oestrogen and its male counterpart – androgen - are steroid hormones that regulate many processes or characteristics that we find in males and females.

Both male and females produce both but more oestrogen is produced in females and more androgens in males.

In conditions like polycystic ovarian syndrome, there appears to be an imbalance of these two hormones. Females produce more androgen than is normal. As a result, they develop characteristics associated with androgens which are:

Excessive hair growth generally on the face following the pattern of male facial hair

Acne and infertility are also found in those with excessive androgens. Those bristly chinned elderly ladies that I remember all too well from my childhood may just have been suffering from a vitamin d deficiency.

Finally, skin pigmentation occurs as a result of excessive androgen.

Thus, if you have:

Acne/infertility

Rotund belly

Hirsutism – the bearded ladies associated with circuses most certainly had excessive androgen levels

Skin pigmentation

Urinary incontinence

High blood pressure due to atherosclerosis narrowing the lumen of the artery

Then it may indicate a deficiency of vitamin D

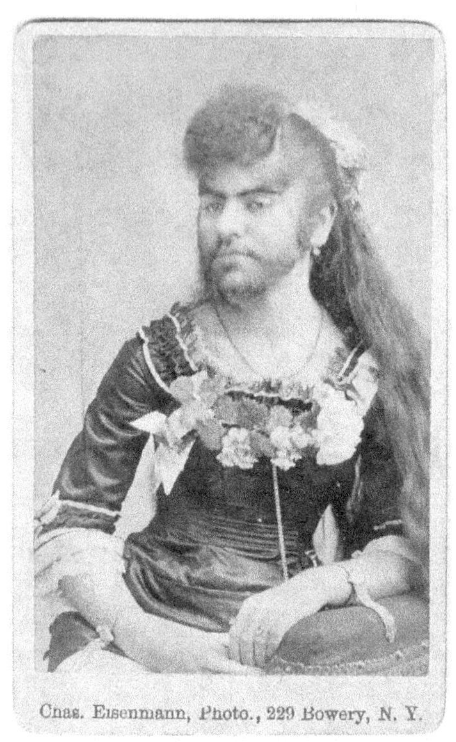

 More pronounced hirsutism in a lady. There are different degrees of it.

Phytoestrogens

Phytoestrogens are plant substances which have structures similar to oestrogen. As such they have similar effects on the body as oestrogen.

Mixed reports on the effectiveness of phytoestrogens are very common. Maybe this could be attributed to menopausal symptoms occurring due to some other nutritional deficiency; maybe results are influenced by each individual's unique intestinal bacteria and its ability to metabolise to therapeutic substances.

Some phytoestrogens appear to be more likely to make a difference than others. There are many phytoestrogens which include:

Soy, lentils and legumes

Coumestans from red clover and bean sprouts

Lignans from grains like flaxseed and other cereal grains

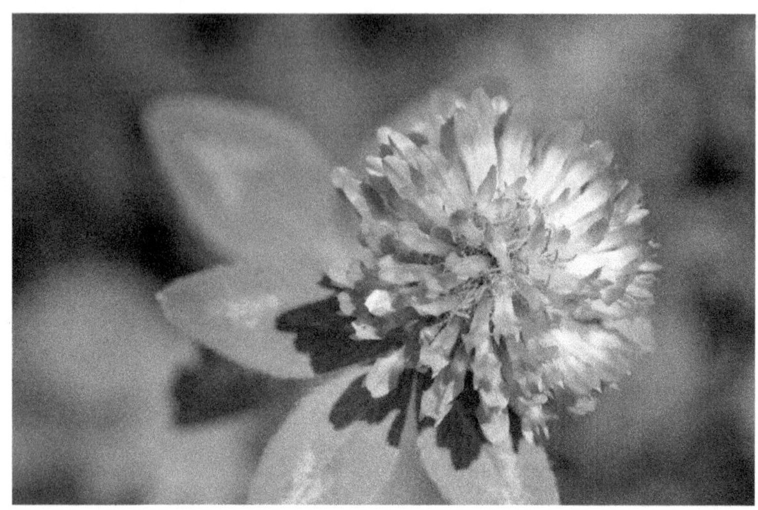

Red clover is a phytoestrogen

It was the isoflavones that appeared to improve menopausal symptoms such as vaginal dryness and hot flashes, so such a systemic impact appears to evidence that urinary symptoms, due to low oestrogen levels, will also improve. Nevertheless, the benefit does not appear to be highly significant.

Adequate Zinc is also needed; as an adaptogen it helps to moderate hormones like oestrogen, progesterone and cortisol due to excesses or insufficiency of them.

Storage of zinc in the body is limited. No more than 24 hours of the average individual's needs is stored. Diuretics will flush zinc away rapidly and antacids prevent zinc from being absorbed. Individuals on iron tablets will not absorb zinc well and those on high copper diets will find that zinc absorption is compromised.

Going on a diet in order to beat the potential weight gain that is associated with the menopause, appears counterproductive. It is no surprise that people on calorie reducing diets tend to put even more weight on once they've finished dieting, Perhaps, we should call these diets 'nutrient deficiency diets.'

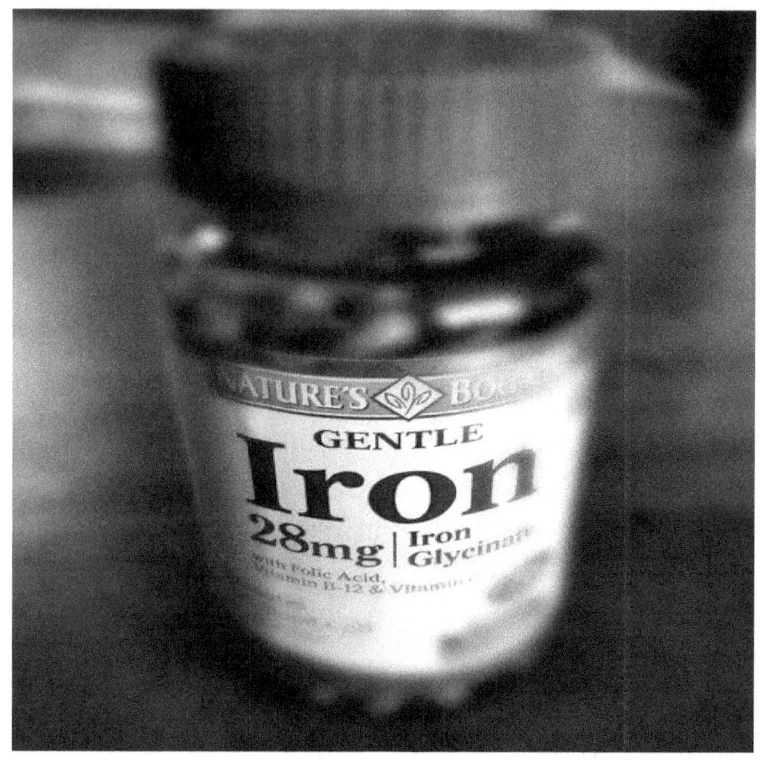

Iron prevents the absorption of zinc

Sometimes, in order to understand what is likely cause of urinary incontinence, it helps to look at medication which is prescribed to address this condition. Every medication has an active site which interacts with, and impacts metabolic pathways. Understanding this helps find more natural treatments with a similar, but more gentle action.

Oxybutynin, a commonly prescribed medication.

A commonly prescribed medication is Ditropan also known as oxybutynin. Ditropan is an anticholinergic medication prescribed for those with an overactive bladder which includes frequency and urgency.

Anticholinergics block the action of acetylcholine, a substance that is involved in movement. For example, sufficient acetylcholine is required to stimulate bowel movements.

Acetylcholine is found in the synapses of the peripheral and central nervous system. Ditropan works by blocking acetylcholine from attaching to its receptors in nerve cells.

Ditropan is useful for those experiencing bladder spasms due to its ability to calm the smooth muscle of the bladder. Bladder spasms are a side effect of indwelling catheters.

Ditropan is well absorbed and delays the feeling of the need to void urine. It can be prescribed in doses of 5mg, 10mg and 15mg with the lesser amounts being given to children as Ditropan can be prescribed for children 5 years and upwards.

It is given as a once a day treatment or up to 4 times a day, depending on need. However, it is not recommended that more than 20mg is taken daily.

Anticholinergic drugs do not come without negative side effects. They are, for example, not recommended for elderly patients. The benefits must outweigh the risks. So, what are the risks?

Ditropan is not generally recommended for pregnant women as there is an increased risk to the developing embryo/foetus. However, there haven't been that many studies on the impact of Ditropan on pregnant women.

Ditropan is not contraindicated for breastfeeding mums. However, the expectation is that babies should be monitored for

Poor feeding habit

Constipation as anticholinergic medications slow down movement,

Fewer wet nappies

Sleepiness (anticholinergic medications if they enter breast milk will cause drowsiness)

There are many adverse effects which include:

Dizziness

Constipation

Dry mouth and mucous tissues which could enhance the transmission of infective agents as the natural moist barrier is no longer.

 Blurred vision and dry eyes

Urinary retention

indigestion

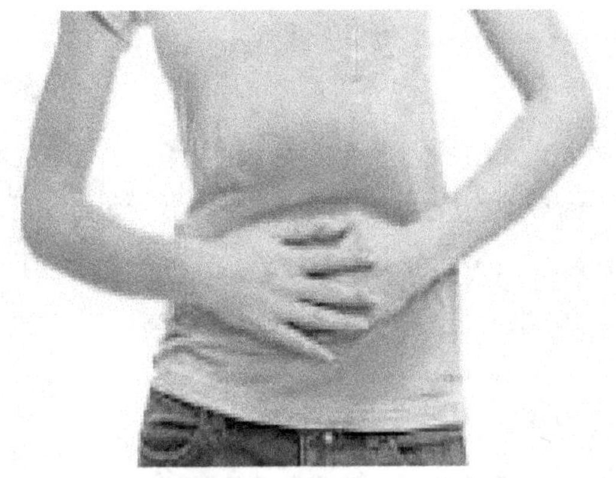

Indigestion is a common symptom of anticholinergic medication

Drowsiness may be so marked that the patient is advised not to drive or use machinery.

There are also reports of psychotic behaviour in those on this medication although this is reported to be rare.

Angioedema of the face, tongue, lips and throat may occur in susceptible people.

Ditropan and the risk of dementia

A number of studies have evidence that taking Ditropan in older patients is a risk factor for dementias, the very group that is more likely to take Ditropan.

A 2009 study entitled **Drugs with anticholinergic properties, cognitive decline, and dementia in an elderly population; the 3-city study** is evidence of this

The study made comparison of both men and women who were over the age of 65. Cognitive decline was evident but took different forms.

In the women, cognitive decline took the form of decline in verbal fluency as well as global cognitive functioning. On the other hand, in men, visual memory was impaired as well as executive function where executive function is taken to mean the mental processes that enable us to plan, remember instructions, focus and multi task.

Executive function helps us to filter out distractions, control impulses, be able to prioritise task and be able to achieve planned goal directed aims.

Those where there is a known familial risk for cognitive disorders like Alzheimer's and Parkinson's disease should avoid these prescription drugs and consider other forms of treatment for incontinence.

Another later study, undertaken in 2015 also had similar results. In this study, 3400 participants over the age of 65 years who showed no sign of dementia at the beginning of the study, were followed up every two years.

The results showed that higher cumulative doses of any anticholinergic drug was linked to an increased risk for dementia. In particular, doses of 5mg daily for a period of 3 years was specifically noted as having a far greater risk for dementia.

In spite of these concerns – also reflected in later studies, over 25% of the over 65's takes an anticholinergic medicine to address urinary incontinence, this is spite of the fact that newer medications do not have this effect or it is attenuated somewhat.

However, Ditropan is by far the cheapest drug.

Describing the impact on cognitive decline, it was stated that there was a 50% increase in dementia cases if more than 1095 doses were taken in a period of a decade.

Currently, there are lawsuits out from those who have suffered from symptoms of dementia.

Concerning is that in 1998 a small study showed that oxybutynin   caused 'significant cognitive effects on 7 out of 15 cognitive measure; this in less than two hours since it was administered.

Although the recommendations were that those on oxybutynin should be monitored, it does not really help those who have taken it because such cognitive impairment has not been shown to be reversible.

Considering the above, Ditropan does not appear safe for long term use but in terms of the independence that it offers, it clearly has benefits. People with bladder problems tend to plan trips around accessible toilets which can work until you turn up at a supermarket to find that the disability toilet is out of order yet again.

So, are there natural alternatives to oxybutynin; ones which will reduce the spasms which are a part of an overactive bladder? In a paper entitled

Alternatives to oxybutynin

Glycine, the smallest of the amino acids, packs a powerful punch in ameliorating most of the problems found with incontinence, in both men and women.

Glycine can be bought in crystalline form. It looks like sugar and is sweet like sugar. As it has inhibitory properties, it can reduce anxiety and aid sleep.

It's use in urinary incontinence relies on the fact that it inhibits the nerve impulses in the spinal cord which are responsible for the micturition reflex.

It has also been noted that men with BPH have lower levels than those who do not have BPH.

Further, the lower the glycine levels the more the bladder contraction pressure and their frequency occurs.

A 4-week study investigated whether 3g of glycine twice daily or glucose in twenty patients delivered greater improvements in areas such as:

Cardiovascular function

Bladder pain

Sleep quality

Greater improvement was found in the group taking glycine.

Due to the small sample group, a larger study was undertaken. There was a high drop-out rate in the glucose group as there was little impact on symptoms. However, those on the glycine stayed until the end as there was symptomatic improvement.

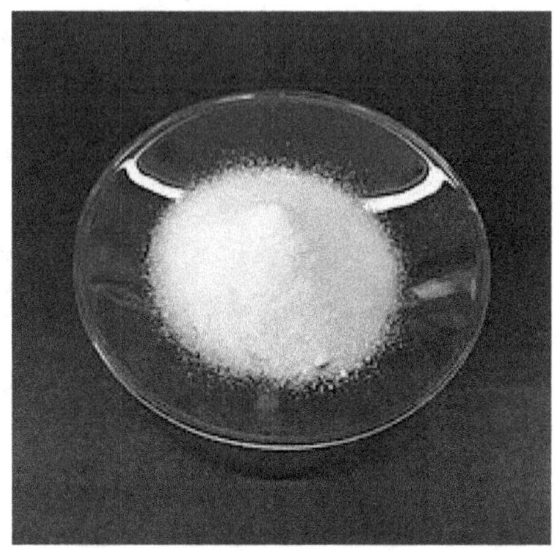

Glycine, the smallest of the amino acids but invaluable in incontinence issues

How long did it take before the results of glycine supplementation were felt?

It took approximately 2 months of oral glycine to improve symptoms of:

Nocturia

Urgency

Frequency

Bladder pain

As an unexpected side effect, blood pressure reduction occurred.

In healthy rats given glycine, bladder contractions occurred less than without the glycine.

There are plenty of sources of glycine so it is possible, with this knowledge, to increase intake sufficiently to address a multiplicity of bladder issues.

Sources of glycine include:

All meats especially those that form a gelatinous mass in the gravy, when cooked.

Fish, especially canned salmon

Hard cheese

Legumes, seeds and peanuts

Quinoa

Eggs

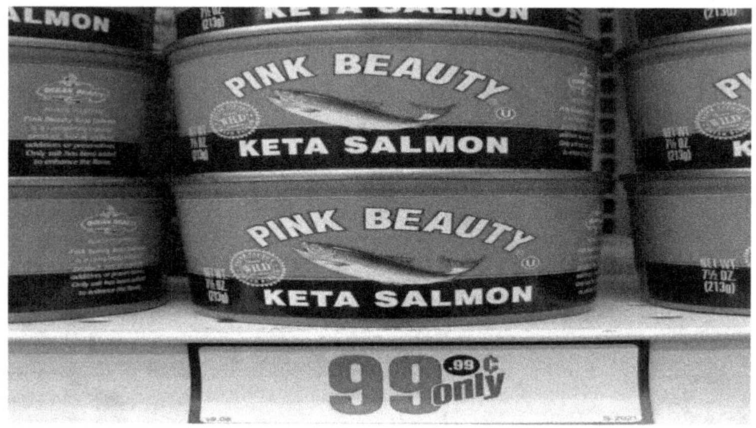

canned salmon contains good amounts of glycine

Finally, glycine is required to prevent the onset of chronic inflammation.

Approximately 2mg of glycine is produced within the body daily but the ageing process will reduce the amount synthesised.

Gelatine, collagen powder and glycine can be added to soups, stews, smoothies. A teaspoon of glycine will adequately sweeten a large mug of tea or coffee and without raising blood sugar levels.

However, 5mg is probably the highest amount that should be taken supplementally and where possible, glycine should be obtained from food. Salmon, for example, contains about 1.4mg glycine in 100g of canned salmon.

If glycine, as an inhibitory amino acid, is able to offer so many benefits for troubling bladder symptoms, are there are other inhibitory amino acids which are able to offer some relief? We shall now turn our attention to tryptophan.

In a paper entitled, *Urinary hesitancy with therapeutic doses of L-tryptophan* by T N Rubin the abstract provides a good overview of the role that tryptophan plays in alleviating incontinence. It is reproduced below.

Note: the doxepin is a tricyclic anti-depressant

L-tryptophan, a precursor of serotonin, in doses of 4 to 5 g/d, has been found to be effective in increasing sleep time, reducing sleep latency, and reducing the number of awakenings. In this report, L-tryptophan 4-6 g/d was administered, along with niacinamide 100 mg and pyridoxine 50 mg, for sleep. Two days after starting L-tryptophan, the patient reported difficulty in voiding. Medications with known anticholinergic activity were selectively discontinued during the patient's hospital course. Seven days after the last dose of L-tryptophan, improvement was noted in the patient's urinary status. Prior to discharge, doxepin was restarted and titrated up to 150 mg/d without a recurrence of urinary problems.

The point to note is that tryptophan did not have to be taken permanently.

Tryptophan is also, like glycine, able to alleviate pain, aid sleep and reduce spasms.

Individuals need about 5mg for ever kilogram of body weight.

Sources of tryptophan are numerous and include:

Animal sources of protein such as meat, fish, eggs, dairy with turkey breast particularly high in tryptophan

Plant sources such as seeds and grains, mushrooms, peas and beans and legumes

Tryptophan can be obtained in powder form or tablet form. It would be especially helpful for those who suffer from nocturia giving people the first good night's sleep that they've had for a long time. However, it can extend your sleep time so if you have to be up early it may not be the first treatment to try.

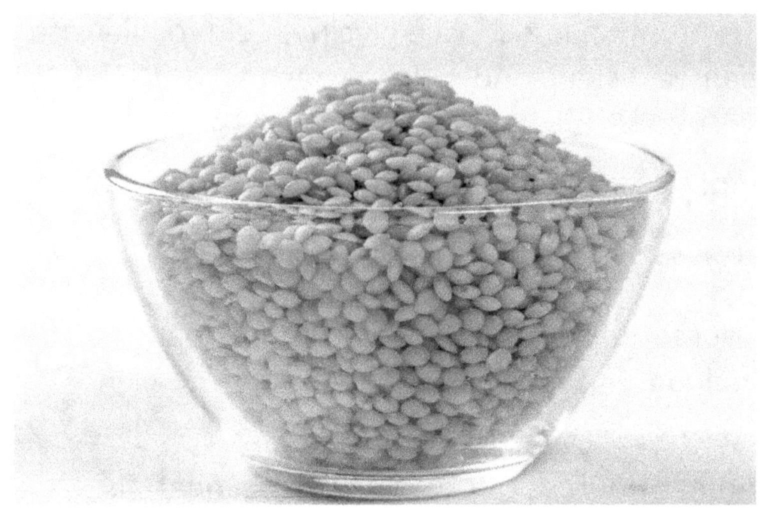

Lentils are a good source of tryptophan.

 In 1989 a patent was developed to treat urinary problems, which included tryptophan. Tryptophan was given in conjunction with another amino acid known as methionine.

Methionine is able to acidify urine and, as such is able to prevent and treat infections of the urinary tract. Lowering acidity helps prevent bacteria from sticking to the bladder wall. In fact, L-methionine is perfect for correcting and treating chronic infection of the urinary tract.

Methionine is able to treat bladder stones and does help to prevent struvite crystals from being formed.

Struvite crystals are a form of kidney stone which has occurred due to an infection so sometimes they are called 'infection stones.' They are composed of magnesium ammonium phosphate.

Methionine is also able to treat gallstones.

Methionine is a sulphur containing amino acid. It is found in similar foods to that in which glycine is found with oats containing much more methionine than other grains.

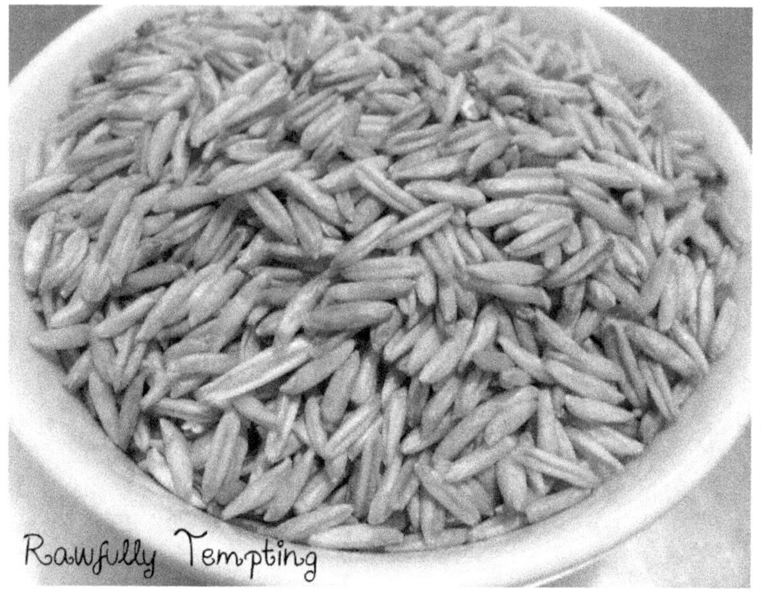

Oats, raw or otherwise, are full of the amino acid, methionine which helps acidify urine thus preventing bacteria from sticking to the bladder walls.

Eating porridge on a regular basis is a wise choice for those who regularly suffer from urinary tract infections. Taken with a glass of fresh orange juice will be beneficial as orange juice is also acidic and the vitamin C has antibacterial properties in itself.

The three amino acids – glycine, tryptophan and methionine are superior to prescription medication in many ways but surely the main benefit is that they are not a risk factor for cognitive decline, are able to be obtained without a prescription and most importantly do work.

The body has always been geared up to run on vitamins and minerals, fats, protein and carbohydrates; it works more than adequately on those substances but any deficiency will result in some symptom such as pain or fatigue or the bladder playing up. No amount of prescription medication can replace the correct nutritional substances for they are bespoke and the perfect remedy for whatever is ailing a person.

The trick is not to run to the GP and expect a prescription to treat an ailment, the trick is to examine the symptoms and diet and find out where there is insufficiency of one or more nutrients and replace those.

It is quite common to find that there are a number of nutritional deficiencies; these appear to be increasing in society all the time with common ones being:

Magnesium

Vitamin C

Vitamin D

Vitamin B1

Zinc

When you take zinc, as an example, it has over 400 functions in the body which if compromised will have a knock on effect into other metabolic pathways. One nutrient deficiency can impact any other setting off a chain reaction of seemingly unrelated symptoms.

How symptoms of conditions impact us differs. Some cause pain or discomfort, others like incontinence impact the quality of life as sufferers tend not to want to wander far from home. Further, any urinary tract infections are painful so that any desire to socialise dissipates.

Getting an appointment with a GP is becoming increasingly more difficult; prescription drugs are, in themselves, often dangerous, so informed consent means knowing what the alternatives are because if you are in pain and discomfort and you are not aware of alternative treatments then it is highly likely that you will choose something inappropriate but that would give you some relief.

Nutritional medicine is not always the fastest at alleviating symptoms – although sometimes it can work in seconds – but it comes as a therapeutic substance that your body recognises and prefers and without the very troubling side effects that prescription and over the counter medications inherently carry.

Urinary Tract Infections

Background

Urinary tract infections (URI's) are very common in females due to their shorter length of urethra compared to men. This enables bacteria to travel more quickly and more easily to the bladder. Women are particularly susceptible during pregnancy, after sex and post menopause. Although antibiotics can be effective, antibiotic resistance is always a concern as is actually being able to get an appointment when you need one. UTI's are painful and debilitating and, if allowed to continue, can spread to the kidneys.

Approximately 50% of women will experience a UTI at least once in their lifetime. Others appear to have them regularly which affects their quality of life and often their relationships.

Some of the UTI's may be due to abnormalities of the urinary tract and while this is not the scope of this book the natural remedies may prevent or cut down the need for antibiotics.

UTI's are mainly bacterial in origin but other infective agents such as viruses and fungi may also be responsible. Uncomplicated UTI's are always due to an infective agent while complicated UTI's will have some underlying structural abnormality which compounds the problem. The most common bacteria is that of *Escherichia coli* and it pops up in hospitals as well as communities.

You would think that regular and effective urine flow would dislodge bacteria from the bladder walls but bacteria adapt to their environment and produce adhesion cells on their surface. Once attached they produce other substances designed to enable them to invade the tissue. One such substance is haemolysin which targets and kills immune system cells.

Dead immune system cells end up as pus in the urine and it is these that the GP is looking for when they dipstick urine.

Bacteria have their defences and we have our, the battle being fought will be won on whether our lifestyles have supported a good immune response.

Urinary pathogens can invade host cells and divide inside our own cells. Hidden –temporarily – from our immune system cells they will divide. This hidden colony will provide the next infection that comes along when the conditions are right.

Vitamin D sufficiency enables both the innate (general defence) and acquired immune system (specialist crack troops) to be activated and this is important in controlling any infection.

However, just as colonisation is a prerequisite for the next infection this can be inhibited by our own microbiota such as Lactobacillus spp (often associated with that cultured in yogurt) and *Staphylococcus epidermis.*

It's important to remove the vulnerability factors which increase the risk for UTI's. Bladder gravel and kidney stones provide surfaces for bacteria to cling to which allows for easier colonisation.

Other avoidable vulnerabilities are a poorly functioning immune system due to poor nutritional choices which must surely be the most common cause of UTI's.

Yes, there are risk factors such as:

Pregnancy

Menopause

Catheter use

Sexual relations (the recommendation is to urinate after to flush any potential infective agents out).

But extra precaution to avoid the susceptibility to infection is of paramount importance and should not be skipped.

Although antibiotics tend to work for most people with Trimethoprim one of the most popular to be prescribed with nitrofurantoin a popular second, a small percentage of patients will not respond to them or, if they do, the ability of the bacteria to hide in human host cells gives them the advantage of recurring when it is safe for them to do so.

If antibiotic resistance has occurred then antibiotics like Co-amoxiclav or cephalexin may be prescribed; the latter usually reserved for pregnant women .

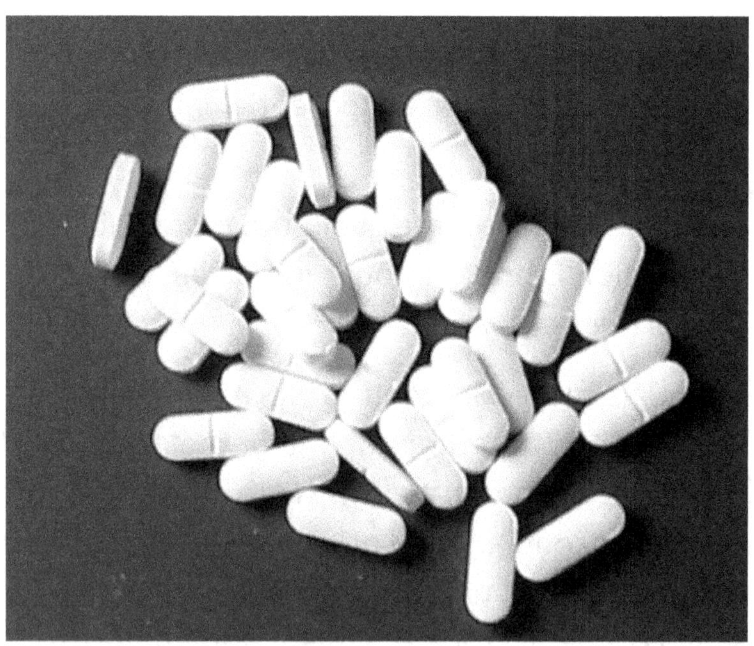

Co-amoxiclav, often used in stubborn cases of infection.

However, UTI's are rife and you have to ask yourself 'where do you go' when UTI's still abound and the antibiotic that did work, although only temporarily, no longer does so.

It has not been fully taken on board that vitamins and minerals do not lose their potency. Bacteria, fungi and viruses do not develop resistance to them so should we not be harnessing the powerful of the substances that our bodies naturally use?

Herbs contain many useful substances. For example, **berberine** helps prevent the adhesion of bacteria to the bladder epithelium

Terpenoids are found in plants such as:

Beer and hops

Eucalyptus

Cinnamon, and other spices

Tomatoes

But this is by no means a definitive list.

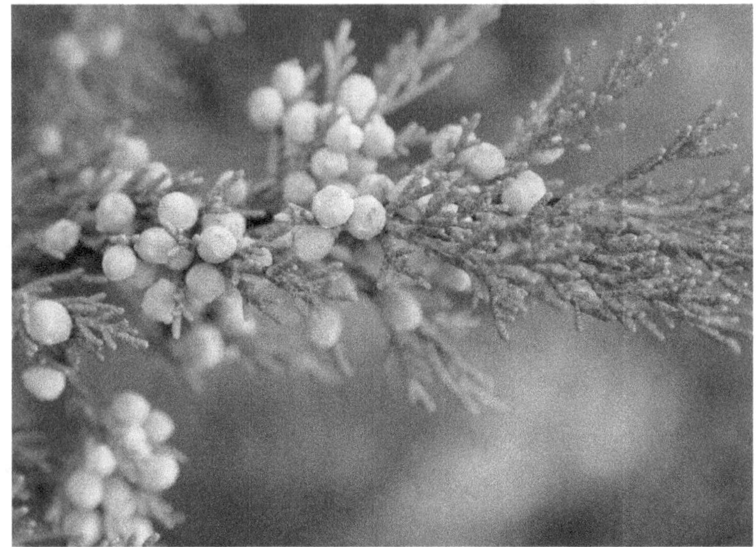

Juniper has remarkable properties when it comes to treating UTI's.

Uva Ursi is able to convert to a substance called hydroquinone which is a direct antimicrobial agent.

The **Juniper** has superior antimicrobial efficacy with the berries and leaves used for making tea. However, juniper does contain highly volatile compounds and so should not be considered as a permanent therapeutic alternative medication.

Cranberry is known to prevent E coli from attaching to the bladder wall. Some people find it effective and others don't. Maybe the latter have a different type of infection.

Cinnamon

Cinnamon has long been known for its antibacterial activities in addition to its antioxidant effects. It is especially useful in being able to inhibit the formation of biofilm which tends to form on catheters.

Small amounts of cinnamon are good; a little sprinkle on the top of coffee, for example, but too much is counterproductive and there are many other herbs and spices which can be used as additions to cinnamon in treating UTI's.

Although I cannot name all the herbs and spices which can be used therapeutically to treat UTI's I will finish off with the humble nettle because it is a plant that can be obtained just about everywhere. There is no point in me extolling the virtue of certain plants if they are impossible to source.

Nettles have so many uses including:

The treatment of kidney stones,

UTI's due to it antibacterial activity against both Gram negative and Gram positive bacteria.

Can be used as a diuretic which would help flush pathogens out of the body

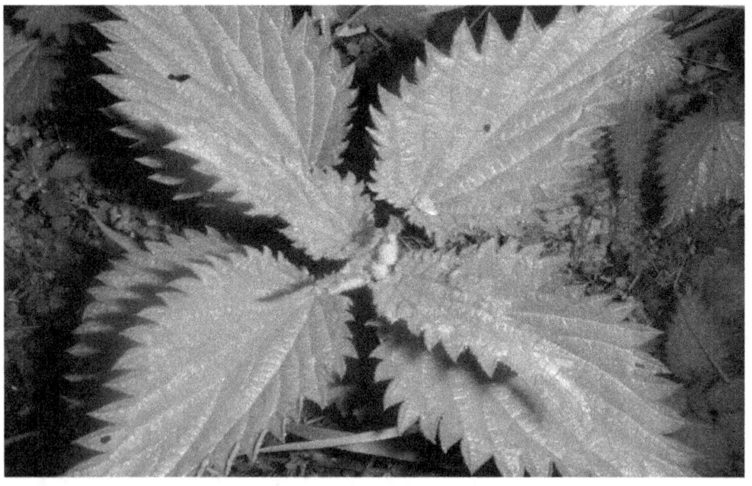

Nettles have a wide range of efficacy against bacteria

The role of nutrition therapy in the prevention and treatment of UTIs. The ingredients with the related mechanism of action(s) are also described.

Most vitamins will have their own specific impact of various aspects of UTI's. I intend to skip over this fairly quickly as this has been dealt with in earlier chapters.

Vitamin A – protects epithelial barrier and helps to prevent renal scarring.

Vitamin C – produces nitric oxide, is a powerful antimicrobial and antioxidant. It has the ability to acidify thus producing a hostile environment for bacteria in which to thrive.

Vitamin D helps restore the lining of the bladder as well as activating the innate and acquired immune system

Selenium is required in the synthesis of selenoproteins which contain cysteine. They are important in initiating and maintaining an immune response.

D-mannose is a simple sugar which is found in fruit and vegetables as well as coffee beans and guar gums. It is also produced endogenously from glucose and helps the proliferation of good bacteria in the gut.

The use of citrate salts in UTI's works by alkalising the urine. Bacteria can only flourish within a narrow range of pH so acidifying through the use of vitamin C or alkalising it via citrate salts prevents bacteria from taking hold.

Zinc deficiency is often found where infectious diseases flourish.

Selenium helps prevent biofilms which are just colonies of bacteria which form a sticky protective film around themselves.

Selenium is known to have two analogues. L-proline and L-cystine which have efficacy in treating UTI's.
It is relatively easy to become deficient in selenium since plants cannot take it up in selenium depleted soils. Two brazil nuts should provide all the selenium that you need daily but this would depend on if the brazil nuts were grown in selenium rich soil.

Copper is known to be a superior antibacterial agent. Copper absorption is inhibited when the diet contains too much iron and zinc. Copper does inhibit E. coli colonisation.

It can be understood that preventing the need for antibiotics by adherence to principles of good nutritional intake is judicious. Once a UTI has taken hold, it evidences that the body's own defences have been breached and this first and foremost needs attention. Every nutrient works in a slightly different way to another nutrient and all help to repair any damage caused by deficits as well as maintain the general defences the body is more than capable of undertaking.

Every person will have their own specific set of genetic vulnerabilities so that some people may never be troubled by UTI's but be more susceptible to respiratory infection. Thus all people may vary their diets from the norm for that culture, in order to deal with such differences. Often this is undertaken without even thinking about it and 'just knowing' what makes them feel worse or better.

In the end, pharmaceuticals have a very limited range of therapeutic interventions and many of these have troubling side effects. Natural alternatives which work with nutrients that the body has always run on, work best, support the immune system and come with very few, if any negative side effects

Table: Nutrients and Their Roles in UTI Prevention

Nutrient / Compound	Mechanism	How It Supports Urinary Health
Vitamin A	Maintains epithelial integrity	Strengthens bladder lining and reduces vulnerability to infection

Nutrient / Compound	Mechanism	How It Supports Urinary Health
Vitamin C	Antioxidant; acidifies urine; supports nitric oxide	Creates hostile environment for bacteria; supports immune defence
Vitamin D	Regulates immune responses; supports tissue repair	Helps restore bladder lining and immune readiness
Zinc	Immune cell function	Supports effective immune response to bacteria
Selenium	Antioxidant; prevents biofilms	Reduces bacterial protection mechanisms
Copper	Natural antibacterial	Inhibits E. coli growth
D-mannose	Reduces bacterial adhesion	Helps prevent bacteria attaching to bladder wall
Citrate salts	Alkalise urine	Disrupts bacterial growth conditions
Magnesium	Neuromuscular support	Helps reduce bladder irritability
Polyphenols	Anti-adhesion and antioxidant	May reduce bacterial attachment and inflammation

Collagen, Connective Tissue, and the Changing Understanding of Incontinence

Urinary incontinence affects millions of people, yet the underlying biology is rarely explained in a way that feels both understandable and hopeful. Much of the public conversation focuses on pelvic floor muscles alone, but continence depends just as much on the **connective tissues** that support the bladder, urethra, and pelvic organs. These tissues are built largely from collagen. When collagen weakens, stretches, or degrades with age, childbirth, hormonal changes, or illness, the pelvic floor loses its structural integrity. This can make leakage more likely during movement, coughing, lifting, or even at rest.

Recent research has begun to explore whether **collagen supplementation**, particularly **marine collagen peptides**, may help strengthen these tissues from within. While the science is still developing, early findings are promising and align with what we know about how collagen behaves in the body.

The Role of Collagen in Pelvic Support

Collagen is the most abundant protein in the human body. It forms the scaffolding that gives tissues their shape, strength, and elasticity. In the pelvis, collagen is essential for:

- **The fascia** that supports the bladder and urethra
- **The ligaments** that maintain organ position
- **The connective tissue** that anchors pelvic floor muscles
- **The urethral wall**, which requires firmness to maintain closure pressure

When collagen fibres weaken, the pelvic floor cannot provide the same level of support. This is one reason why incontinence becomes more common with age, menopause, and connective-tissue changes.

Why Marine Collagen Peptides Are of Interest

Marine collagen is derived from fish skin and scales. It contains **smaller peptides** than bovine or porcine collagen, which makes it easier for the body to absorb and use. This higher bioavailability is one reason researchers are exploring its potential benefits for connective-tissue repair.

Once absorbed, collagen peptides may:

- Stimulate **new collagen synthesis**

- Improve **tissue elasticity**
- Support **extracellular matrix turnover**
- Strengthen **muscle–tendon interfaces**
- Enhance **hydration** of connective tissues

These mechanisms are relevant to continence because they influence the tissues that help keep the bladder neck and urethra supported.

What Current Research Suggests

Early studies have examined collagen in combination with pelvic floor exercises and magnesium. A **double-blind, randomised pilot clinical trial** found that a supplement containing collagen and magnesium, combined with pelvic floor muscle training, improved symptoms in women with urinary incontinence.

A **systematic review** of urinary incontinence, pelvic floor training, and collagen also highlighted collagen's importance in pelvic support and its interaction with pelvic diaphragm muscle fibres.

Although some research has focused on **injectable collagen** as a bulking agent for stress incontinence, which is a different approach, it reinforces the principle that collagen contributes meaningfully to urethral support.

A more recent **pilot evaluation** again found improvements when collagen and magnesium supplementation were combined with pelvic floor exercises.

These studies vary in design and strength, but together they point toward a consistent theme: **collagen plays a structural role in continence**, and supporting collagen production may help improve symptoms for some people.

A Case Study

Case Study: "M." – Gradual Improvement Through Connective-Tissue Support

M. is a 62-year-old retired teacher who experienced mild stress incontinence, especially when lifting shopping bags or walking briskly. She began taking a daily marine collagen peptide supplement for joint comfort. Over six to eight weeks, she noticed:

- Fewer leakage episodes
- A greater sense of pelvic stability
- Improved confidence during physical activity

She had not been aware of any research linking collagen to continence. Her GP later explained that improved connective-tissue integrity could plausibly contribute to better urethral support. This case illustrates how systemic collagen support may influence continence without implying universal results.

Vitamin D and Continence

Vitamin D is essential for muscle strength, neuromuscular signalling, and inflammation control. Low levels are associated with weaker pelvic floor muscles and increased risk of incontinence. Adequate vitamin D may:

- Improve pelvic floor muscle contraction
- Reduce inflammation in pelvic tissues
- Support overall musculoskeletal function

Including vitamin-D-rich foods can complement collagen's connective-tissue benefits.

Tables for Clarity

Mechanisms Linking Collagen to Continence

Mechanism	Effect on Pelvic Floor
Strengthening connective tissue	Better bladder neck and urethral support
Enhanced collagen turnover	Repair of stretched pelvic fascia
High bioavailability of marine peptides	Faster incorporation into tissues
Improved muscle–tendon interface	More effective pelvic floor muscle action

Types of Collagen

Type	Source	Bioavailability	Notes
Marine	Fish skin/scales	High	Small peptides, well absorbed

Type	Source	Bioavailability	Notes
Bovine	Cow hide/bone	Moderate	Widely available
Porcine	Pig skin	Moderate	Similar to bovine

Tables

Collagen Mechanisms and Their Relevance to Continence

Mechanism	What It Does	Why It Matters for Continence
Strengthening connective tissue	Improves tensile strength of fascia and ligaments	Better support for bladder neck and urethra
Enhanced collagen turnover	Encourages repair of stretched or weakened tissues	May reduce stress incontinence
High bioavailability of marine peptides	Faster absorption and utilisation	More efficient tissue support

Mechanism	What It Does	Why It Matters for Continence
Improved muscle–tendon interface	Supports pelvic floor muscle function	Helps muscles contract more effectively
Increased tissue hydration	Improves elasticity	Supports urethral closure pressure

Types of Collagen and Their Features

Type	Source	Bioavailability	Notes
Marine collagen	Fish skin/scales	High	Small peptides, well absorbed
Bovine collagen	Cow hide/bone	Moderate	Common and affordable
Porcine collagen	Pig skin	Moderate	Similar to bovine

Nutrients That Support Pelvic Floor Health

Nutrient	Role	Why It Helps
Marine collagen peptides	Tissue repair	Supports connective-tissue strength
Vitamin D	Muscle function	Low levels linked to pelvic floor weakness

Nutrient	Role	Why It Helps
Magnesium	Neuromuscular signalling	May reduce bladder over activity
Omega-3	Anti-inflammatory	Supports tissue healing
Protein	Muscle maintenance	Helps pelvic floor strength

Ten Additional Recipes (with Method + Why They're Beneficial)

1) Collagen-Enriched Golden Milk

Ingredients:
Marine collagen powder, turmeric, ginger, cinnamon, honey, warm milk (dairy or fortified plant milk).

Method:
Warm the milk gently. Whisk in collagen, turmeric, ginger, and cinnamon. Sweeten lightly.

Why beneficial:
Collagen supports connective tissue; turmeric may reduce inflammation.

2) Vitamin-D Mushroom Soup

Ingredients:
Sun-exposed mushrooms, onion, garlic, vegetable stock, thyme, a splash of cream.

Method:
Sauté onion and garlic. Add mushrooms and thyme. Pour in stock, simmer, blend, finish with cream.

Why beneficial:
Sun-exposed mushrooms naturally contain vitamin D, supporting muscle function.

---

3) Salmon and Collagen Fishcakes

Ingredients:
Cooked salmon, mashed potato, parsley, lemon zest, egg, marine collagen powder.

Method:
Mix ingredients, shape into patties, pan-fry until golden.

Why beneficial:
Salmon provides vitamin D and omega-3; collagen adds connective-tissue support.

---

4) Spinach and Sardine Toast

Ingredients:
Wholegrain toast, sardines in olive oil, wilted spinach, lemon.

Method:
Toast bread, top with warm sardines and spinach, squeeze lemon.

Why beneficial:
Sardines are rich in vitamin D, calcium, and omega-3.

---

5) Collagen-Boosted Lentil Stew

Ingredients:
Red lentils, carrots, celery, tomatoes, cumin, marine collagen.

Method:
Simmer lentils with vegetables and spices. Stir collagen in at the end.

Why beneficial:
Lentils provide magnesium and plant protein; collagen supports tissue repair.

---

6) Egg Muffins with Vitamin-D Mushrooms

Ingredients:
Eggs, chopped mushrooms, spinach, cheese, pepper.

Method:
Mix ingredients, pour into muffin tins, bake until set.

Why beneficial:
Eggs and mushrooms both contribute vitamin‑D;
protein supports pelvic floor strength.

---

7) Collagen Berry Chia Pudding

Ingredients:
Chia seeds, milk, collagen powder, berries, vanilla.

Method:
Mix chia, milk, collagen, and vanilla. Refrigerate
overnight. Top with berries.

Why beneficial:
Collagen supports connective tissue; chia provides
magnesium and omega-3.

---

8) Mackerel and Avocado Salad

Ingredients:
Smoked mackerel, avocado, mixed leaves, lemon, olive oil.

Method:
Flake mackerel, toss with leaves and avocado, dress with lemon and oil.

Why beneficial:
Mackerel is high in vitamin D and omega-3; avocado adds healthy fats.

---

9) Collagen-Infused Vegetable Broth

Ingredients:
Carrots, celery, onion, garlic, herbs, marine collagen.

Method:
Simmer vegetables in water for 45 minutes. Strain. Stir collagen into the warm broth.

Why beneficial:
A gentle, hydrating way to take collagen; warm fluids may ease pelvic tension.

---

10) Magnesium-Rich Almond and Banana Smoothie

Ingredients:
Banana, almond butter, milk, cinnamon, marine collagen (optional).

Method:
Blend all ingredients until smooth.

Why beneficial:
Almonds provide magnesium, which supports neuromuscular function.

---

11) Collagen-Fortified Oat Porridge

Ingredients:
Oats, milk or water, collagen powder, blueberries, flaxseed.

Method:
Cook oats, stir in collagen, top with berries and flax.

Why beneficial:
Oats and flax support digestion; collagen supports tissue repair.

12) Sunshine Omelette

Ingredients:
Eggs, smoked salmon, chives, mushrooms.

Method:
Sauté mushrooms, add beaten eggs, fold in salmon and chives.

Why beneficial:
Eggs and salmon both contain vitamin D; protein supports pelvic floor strength.

---

13) Collagen-Enhanced Tomato and Basil Soup

Ingredients:
Tomatoes, onion, garlic, basil, stock, collagen.

Method:
Simmer tomatoes with aromatics, blend, stir collagen in before serving.

Why beneficial:
Collagen supports connective tissue; tomatoes provide antioxidants.

---

14) Greek Yoghurt with Seeds and Collagen

Ingredients:
Greek yoghurt, pumpkin seeds, sunflower seeds, collagen, honey.

Method:
Mix collagen into yoghurt, top with seeds and honey.

Why beneficial:
Seeds provide magnesium; yoghurt may be fortified with vitamin D.

---

15) Roasted Mackerel with Lemon and Herbs

Ingredients:
Whole mackerel or fillets, lemon, parsley, olive oil.

Method:
Roast mackerel with lemon slices and herbs until flaky.

Why beneficial:
One of the richest natural sources of vitamin D and omega-3.

- **Berry Collagen Smoothie** — marine collagen powder, blueberries, kefir, flaxseed.
- **Lemon-Ginger Collagen Tea** — marine collagen dissolved in warm water with lemon and ginger.
- **Collagen-Boosted Vegetable Soup** — add unflavoured marine collagen to broth-based soups.

Vitamin-D-Rich Recipes

- **Grilled Salmon with Herbs** — high in vitamin D and omega-3.
- **Mushroom and Spinach Omelette** — mushrooms exposed to sunlight contain meaningful vitamin D.
- **Fortified Yoghurt Parfait** — fortified yoghurt layered with nuts and seeds.

Brain Injury and Continence: Why Neurological Causes Are Often Missed

Every year, large numbers of people experience some form of brain injury—from stroke, concussion, falls, inflammation, infection, or age-related change—and many of these injuries are never formally diagnosed. Mild or moderate injuries often go unnoticed because symptoms may be subtle, delayed, or attributed to ageing, stress, or unrelated health issues. When the regions of the brain involved in bladder awareness, inhibition, or coordination are affected, incontinence can appear without any obvious cause. Because the underlying neurological injury may not be recognised, the incontinence is sometimes treated as a purely bladder or pelvic floor problem, which can lead to incomplete or inappropriate management. A qualified healthcare professional should be consulted for assessment of any new or persistent incontinence, as neurological causes require clinical evaluation.

Diagram: Key Brain Regions Involved in Continence

Caption:
The major brain regions involved in continence. The frontal lobe provides conscious inhibition; the insula and parietal lobe process bladder sensation; the basal ganglia regulate automatic suppression of bladder contractions; the brainstem coordinates the switch between storage and voiding; and the cerebellum fine-tunes pelvic floor responses.

How the Brain Controls Continence

Bladder control depends on a network of brain regions that work together to sense bladder filling, suppress unwanted contractions, and coordinate pelvic floor relaxation when it is time to void. Damage to any part of this network can result in urgency, frequency, or incontinence.

Prefrontal Cortex

- Provides conscious inhibition ("holding on").
- Damage reduces the ability to delay voiding or judge appropriate timing.

Anterior Cingulate Cortex

- Integrates emotional, sensory, and autonomic signals.
- Injury disrupts the ability to coordinate urge with behaviour.

Insular Cortex

- Processes internal sensations, including bladder fullness.
- Damage reduces awareness of filling, leading to unexpected leakage.

Parietal Lobe

- Helps interpret sensory information from the bladder.
- Injury may cause misinterpretation of urgency or reduced sensation.

Basal Ganglia

- Regulate automatic motor patterns and suppress unwanted bladder contractions.
- Damage (e.g., Parkinson's disease) leads to urgency and frequency.

Pontine Micturition Centre (Brainstem)

- Coordinates bladder contraction with sphincter relaxation.

- Damage causes loss of coordinated voiding, overflow, or continuous leakage.

Cerebellum

- Fine-tunes motor responses, including pelvic floor coordination.
- Injury may cause urgency or difficulty contracting the pelvic floor effectively.

Spinal Cord Pathways

- Carry messages between bladder and brain.
- Damage can cause overactivity, underactivity, or loss of voluntary control.

Nutritional Medicine to Support Neural Recovery

Nutritional strategies cannot reverse structural neurological injury, but they can support the biological processes involved in neural repair, inflammation control, and tissue resilience. Persistent or worsening incontinence should be assessed by a qualified healthcare professional.

Omega-3 Fatty Acids

- Support neuronal membrane repair.

- Help modulate neuroinflammation.

B-Vitamins (B1, B6, B9, B12)

- Support myelin maintenance and nerve conduction.
- Contribute to neurotransmitter synthesis involved in bladder signalling.

Choline

- Supports acetylcholine production, essential for bladder–brain communication.
- Helps repair cell membranes.

Magnesium

- Supports neuromuscular signalling.
- May help stabilise overactive bladder pathways.

Vitamin D

- Supports immune regulation and neural tissue health.
- Contributes to pelvic floor muscle function.

Antioxidants (Vitamin C, Vitamin E, Polyphenols)

- Reduce oxidative stress after neural injury.
- Support tissue repair and inflammation resolution.

Selenium and Zinc

- Support immune balance and antioxidant enzymes.
- Contribute to tissue repair and neural resilience.

Protein and Collagen Peptides

- Support repair of connective tissues around the bladder and urethra.
- Provide amino acids needed for healing and muscle maintenance.

Table 1: Brain Regions and Their Role in Continence

Brain Region	Function in Bladder Control	Effect of Damage
Prefrontal cortex	Voluntary inhibition	Urgency, inappropriate voiding
Anterior cingulate cortex	Integrates urge and behaviour	Poor coordination of response
Insular cortex	Sensation of bladder fullness	Reduced awareness, unexpected leakage
Parietal lobe	Interpretation of bladder signals	Misinterpreted urgency or reduced sensation
Basal ganglia	Suppression of unwanted contractions	Frequency, urgency
Pontine micturition centre	Coordinates voiding	Overflow, retention, loss of control
Cerebellum	Fine-tunes pelvic floor responses	Poor coordination, urgency

Brain Region	Function in Bladder Control	Effect of Damage
Spinal pathways	Communication between bladder and brain	Reflexive emptying or loss of control

Table 2: Nutrients Supporting Neural and Bladder Function

Nutrient	Mechanism	Potential Contribution
Omega-3 fatty acids	Membrane repair	Supports neural recovery
B-vitamins	Myelin and nerve signalling	Supports bladder–brain communication
Choline	Neurotransmitter synthesis	Supports signalling pathways
Magnesium	Neuromuscular function	May reduce bladder irritability
Vitamin D	Immune and muscle regulation	Supports neural and pelvic floor health
Selenium	Antioxidant enzyme support	Protects neural tissue

Nutrient	Mechanism	Potential Contribution
Zinc	Immune and tissue repair	Supports recovery processes
Collagen peptides	Connective-tissue support	Supports pelvic floor structures
Vitamin C	Collagen synthesis	Supports tissue repair
Polyphenols	Anti-inflammatory	May reduce neuroinflammation

ALSO BY LYNNE D. M. NOBLE

Dermatology & Autoimmune Skin Conditions

- The Psoriasis Diet
- A Diet for Psoriasis
- Granuloma Annulare: The Complete Nutritional & Lifestyle Guide

Connective Tissue Disorders & Chronic Pain

- The Journey: Living with EDS and Chronic Pain
- The EDS and Hypermobility Syndrome Diet
- Alleviating Symptoms of EDS
- Causes of Weight Gain in EDS
- The EDS Recipe Book

Rheumatology & Autoimmune Joint Disease

- Dietary Strategies for RA: Understanding and Interrupting the Inflammatory Loop
- Osteoarthritis and Pain (Colour Edition)
- Pain: Causes and Treatment of Pain Associated with Fibromyalgia, Arthritis and Soft Tissue
- Uncovering Fibromyalgia (Black & White Edition)
- Uncovering Fibromyalgia (Colour Edition)

Neurology & Neurodegenerative Conditions

- Parkinson's Disease: Dietary Changes That Work
- Multiple Sclerosis Tamed
- Treatment Strategy for Migraine
- Healing Shingles and Neuropathic Pain
- Dietary Deficiencies in Tinnitus and Hearing Impairment
- The Alzheimer's and Vascular Dementia Disease Diet

Endocrine, Hormonal & Metabolic Health

- The Thyroid Diet
- Nutritional Strategies to Correct PCOS and Infertility
- The Metabolic Syndrome Diet
- A Weighty Issue: Obesity — Its Causes and Responses

Cardiovascular & Healthy Ageing

- Why We Live Longer with Higher Cholesterol Levels
- Beat Hypertension Easily Using Nutrition
- Ageing and How to Avoid It

Lymphatic, Lipoedema & Lymphoedema Health

- The Lipoedema Diet
- The Lipoedema Diet: An Exploration of Nutritional Substances That Attenuate the Processes Involved in the Development of Lipoedema
- The Lymphoedema Diet (Black & White Edition)
- The Lymphoedema Diet: Reverse and Repair Lymphatic Damage

Respiratory, Immune & Infectious Disease

- Innate and Adaptive Immunity in Older Adults: PRRs, Cytokines, Nutrition, and Age Related Change
- How Nutrition Shapes Antibodies, Memory Cells, and Long Term Defence
- Calming the Storm Within: A Nutritional and Scientific Guide to Inflammation
- The Master Switch: Using Food and Lifestyle to Support Your Body's Natural Resilience and Repair Pathways
- Treat Infection Naturally
- Journey Through Pneumonia
- Eat to Beat Viral Infections
- The Anti Virus Diet
- The Asthma Diet

Allergy, Intolerance & Digestive Health

- Allergy and Intolerance: A Dietary Response
- The Constipated Carrot: Constipation — Getting to the Bottom of the Problem
- The Constipated Carrot (Black & White Edition)
- The Chocolate Diet (and Why It Works)
- The Silent Gut: Understanding Motility, Signalling and the Hidden Causes of Constipation

Systems Biology, Lifestyle & Environmental Health

- Tap Water and How to Reduce Its Use
- Sleep: Perchance to Dream
- Foraging and Beyond

Emotional Health, Grief & Personal Development

- Effective Treatment for Anxiety, Stress and
  Depression
- A Personal Grief
- A Necessary Sorrow
- IDENTITY: A Self Exploration (Workbook)
- Living in the Overload: A Life Shaped by Parietal Lobe
  Injury

Parenting & Behaviour

- Difficult Children Are Not the Result of Bad
  Parenting: Blame It on Great Aunt Alice!

Cancer & Oncology Nutrition

- Dietary Responses to Cancer

Back Pain & Musculoskeletal Health

- Effective Treatment for Back Pain
- Banish Back Pain Forever

★ Children's Stories

- Fanny and the Gamekeeper's Cottage
- Fanny and Victorian Jack

The Exodus Project

My first introduction to the far reaching impact of The Exodus Project occurred when I was travelling around Cawthorne in one of their buses, visiting gardens. A young lad was happily munching on a sandwich. He looked up briefly, pointed to the driver and said,' He's my second dad, he is,' then he returned to his sandwich without further comment

Such remarks are often very telling and so I arranged to meet Jackie Peel and Martin Sawdon, at the charity's premises in Barnsley. They set up the Exodus Project 20 years ago. They moved into their current premises – a redundant Methodist church - in 2010.

Both Jackie and Martin have been youth workers in their church. Martin worked in housing for the homeless in addition to working in learning disabilities services in institutional settings.

The work that the Exodus Project undertakes is of paramount importance to the communities it serves. These were former mining communities which became disadvantaged after pit-closures. Currently about 400 children attend mid-week activities from Monday to Thursday inclusive. These activities include dance, drama, craft, music, sports and games. In addition, there are weekend camps, cycle treks, outward bound activities, bowling and swimming. The children are taught valuable life skills including how to cook and   bake. It is all about teaching children how to fulfil their potential and learn skills they will be able to pass onto the next generation.

The grounds, once overgrown, have been turned into a play- and camping - ground. A miniature railway is in the process of being installed.

Martin and Jackie have developed a unique model in that The Exodus Project goes beyond dispensing services. They are keen to build up relationships with the whole family and not just the child that attends the mid- week clubs. In addition, once children have reached the age of fourteen, they are invited to help out with the younger groups as junior volunteers. Once they reach the age of eighteen, they become adult volunteers. This   model   provides a constant supply of help from individuals   who have benefitted already from attending such groups.

The   building is large and inviting.   It is decorated with bold colours and has comfy seating. It is a real home from home; a haven for families who have been disadvantaged by the closure of the life force of its community.

Martin and Jackie have clear ideas about how they wish to develop the Exodus Project but the lottery funding which they benefitted from is no longer available. Sadly, they have had to close two of their clubs due to lack of funding. This decision wasn't taken lightly. They do have two charity shops which raises some money and they obtain some funding from outside organisations for the use of their facilities. However, this is clearly not enough to keep their clubs, weekend activities and building going to cater for the ever growing number of children who are benefitting from the work being undertaken here.   Neither does it allow for future development.

Exodus do have a Just Giving page which can be found here if you wish to help further their work https://www.justgiving.com/exodus

In addition, you can keep up with activities on their Facebook page here https://www.facebook.com/search/top/?q=the%20exodus%20project%20barnsley&epa=SEARCH_BOX

Recommended small businesses

https://skinkiss.org.uk/

https://favouritekafei.co.uk/?fbclid=IwAR1pW2OJNWCtFdIpgU7WWp9JQiQDxbBxu4GfzBfr6648snFYFERRYvGW7Ss

My Buy Me a Coffee website can be found here:

https://www.buymeacoffee.com/lynnedmnobl

The site contains a number of protocols as well as current health related topics